Patient, Heal Thyself

ROBERT M.
VEATCH

Patient, Heal Thyself

How the New Medicine Puts the

Patient in Charge

OXFORD
UNIVERSITY PRESS

2009

OXFORD
UNIVERSITY PRESS

Oxford University Press, Inc., publishes works that further
Oxford University's objective of excellence
in research, scholarship, and education.

Oxford   New York
Auckland   Cape Town   Dar es Salaam   Hong Kong   Karachi
Kuala Lumpur   Madrid   Melbourne   Mexico City   Nairobi
New Delhi   Shanghai   Taipei   Toronto

With offices in
Argentina   Austria   Brazil   Chile   Czech Republic   France   Greece
Guatemala   Hungary   Italy   Japan   Poland   Portugal   Singapore
South Korea   Switzerland   Thailand   Turkey   Ukraine   Vietnam

Library of Congress Cataloging-in-Publication Data
Veatch, Robert M.
Patient, heal thyself: how the new medicine puts the patient in charge / Robert M. Veatch.
p.; cm.   Includes bibliographical references.
ISBN 978-0-19-531372-7
1. Medicine--Decision making. 2. Medical ethics. 3. Medical care--United States. I. Title.   [DNLM: 1. Patient
Participation--trends. 2. Delivery of Health Care--trends. 3. Personal Autonomy. 4. Philosophy, Medical.
5. Physician-Patient Relations. W 85 V394p 2008]
R723.5.V43 2008   610--dc22
2008003515

9 8 7 6 5 4 3 2 1

Printed in the United States of America
on acid-free paper

For
Willard Gaylin
Andre E. Hellegers (1926-1979)
Edmund D. Pellegrino
Victor W. Sidel
physicians who have mastered the art of respecting patients
and given them the freedom to heal

Decision making in medicine has long posed an intriguing and complex problem. The technical, scientific issues of diagnosis, prognosis, and treatment raise such complicated, esoteric issues that no ordinary patient could ever master even a fraction of the necessary knowledge. Since ancient times, patients have had to rely on experts—physicians and other health professional experts—to penetrate the thickets of medical science.

At the same time, the expert cannot possibly know or understand the patient's unique beliefs, values, and preferences that are crucial for knowing what serves the patient's interest. Worse, still, as medical professionals become specialized and separate themselves from the broader community of laypeople, in a sense they become alienated from the patient perspective. They think about medical choices differently and choose options based on values that are not shared by others. In fact, the Hippocratic notion of professionalism suggests that by taking an oath, the physician sets himself or herself apart from other citizens. He or she "professes" a set of obligations that require loyalty to the profession. Just as patients cannot think like health professionals, who have been trained to view medicine with a set of concepts and theories unknown to laypeople, so, likewise, physicians and other health professionals lose the capacity to think like the patient.

The male obstetrician who has delivered a thousand babies cannot possibly get into the mind-set of the young woman in labor for the first time. The oncologist who has chosen out of all the thousands of occupations to give his life to fighting cancer and has cared for thousands of patients who have gone on to die cannot think like the frightened, newly diagnosed breast cancer patient who may have many critical responsibilities flash before her when she learns her diagnosis.

Several times a day TV commercials advise people to "ask your doctor" about some drug when the doctor has no idea what the patient's goals and desires are. It is absurd for a man to ask his doctor, of all people, whether Viagra is right for him. If he is going to ask, the first person should be his wife or other partner. Similarly, as we shall see in chapter 2, asking the physician whether diet or drugs is better for high cholesterol makes no sense in the era of the new medicine and rarely escapes my ridicule. Of course, physicians may be able to provide some technical assistance about whether a particular drug could produce an effect the patient desires, but they are not in a position to "prescribe" that the changes the drug will produce are good for the patient. Patients, themselves, will have to take charge of those decisions.

In my 40 years of work in the field of biomedical ethics, my primary concern has been the division of labor between the health professional (primarily the physician) and the layperson (primarily the patient). Medicine is so complex that great specialization and division of labor are necessary to master even one tiny aspect, yet no professional expert can possibly expect to understand and think like the patient whose life hangs in the balance.

Increasingly, as I dealt with issues in bioethics, I felt a tension between the standard way of thinking about medical choices and the way I saw emerging in my thinking and in the new practices in the patient-physician relation. The discovery of intensely ethical choices in certain special areas of medicine—abortion, euthanasia, and gene manipulation, for example—only made the tension worse. Both physicians and laypeople now acknowledge that these special choices required a moral perspective that comes from outside medicine, but then they immediately shifted back to more traditional ways of thinking about more ordinary decisions about asthma, arthritis, or antibiotics. It was as if physicians occasionally had to call time-out from their routine, scientifically based medicine to let patients do their value thing on the special, value-loaded choices.

Many years ago I realized that my understanding of medicine was at odds with normal modern thinking. I began to recognize that literally every medical choice required a value perspective and that the health professional could not claim expertise on that value dimension. Gradually, I have discovered that others are beginning to recognize this as well. They are moving to a "new medicine" in which patients must be in charge of making the calls.

This volume is the culmination of this career-long journey toward what I call a new or postmodern medicine. It is a medicine that had its beginnings in the exciting days of the 1970s when patients first began demanding their right to make medical choices based on their own values. It is a medicine now irreversibly launched as the replacement for what is now old-fashioned modern medicine. It is a medicine that is radically different from modern medicine in the role the layperson must play in medical decision making.

In this volume I bring together my thoughts over the past decades. I make a case that a new medicine is well on its way to emerging and that it is destined to replace modern medicine. It is a medicine that will rely on professional medical expertise as much or more than before for more technical matters of diagnosis, prognosis, and treatment options, but will require a much more active patient in charge of choosing which options are best for his or her own medical decisions. It is a world in which physicians and health professionals will become assistants of patient who will have to take charge and heal themselves.

This manuscript has been in preparation for several years. Some of the ideas have germinated, often in only partially developed form, in articles I have written over the years:

Portions of chapters 3–6 incorporate some parts of "Doctor Does Not Know Best: Why in the New Century Physicians Must Stop Trying to Benefit Patients," *Journal of Medicine and Philosophy* 25, no. 6 (December 2000):701–721, by permission of Oxford University Press.

Portions of chapters 11 and 12 are adapted from "Abandoning Informed Consent," *Hastings Center Report* 25, no. 2 (March–April 1995):5–12, © The Hastings Center. Reprinted with permission.

Portions of chapters 16 and 17 are adapted from "Single Payers and Multiple Lists: Must Everyone Get the Same Coverage in a Universal Health Plan?" *Kennedy Institute of Ethics Journal* 7, no. 2 (1997): 153–169.

Portions of chapters 20 and 21 draw on "Indifference of Subjects: An Alternative to Equipoise in Randomized Clinical Trials," in *Bioethics*, ed. Ellen Frankel Paul, Fred D. Miller, Jr., and Jeffrey Paul, 295–323 (Cambridge: Cambridge University Press, 2002). Reprinted with the permission of Cambridge University Press.

Portions of chapters 23–24 incorporate "Technology Assessment: Inevitably a Value Judgment," in *Getting Doctors to Listen: Ethics and Outcomes Data in Context*, ed. Philip J. Boyle, 180–195 (Washington, DC: Georgetown University Press, 1998) © 1998 by Georgetown

University Press, reprinted with permission; and "Consensus of Expertise: The Role of Consensus of Experts in Formulating Public Policy and Estimating Facts," *The Journal of Medicine and Philosophy* 16 (1991):427–445, by permission of Oxford University Press.

In all of these chapters new material is included and material from articles has been revised and integrated into a coherent account of what I am calling the new medicine.

ACKNOWLEDGMENTS

I have over the years given prominent attention to the individual case. In collaboration with others, I have written six different collections of case studies, some of which have gone through multiple editions. I incorporate some cases in this volume to illustrate the themes I develop. A few of the cases are stories I have told before, particularly in the new edition of *Case Studies in Medical Ethics*, which is also published by Oxford University Press, but all reflect some real-life event that shows how values from outside medicine must shape medical decisions.

I had help from many people in developing the ideas and text for this manuscript. My colleagues at the Kennedy Institute of Ethics have been a continual stimulus for decades. They will recognize some of their input in this volume. The professional librarians of the National Reference Center for Bioethics Literature, the Kennedy Institute's library, are a rich resource that any academic researcher would treasure. Their knowledge of the field and its literature has been enormously helpful, as has been the support of Linda Powell, Moheba Hanif, and Sally Schofield. Alexander Curtis and Traviss Cassidy have read large portions of the manuscript and offered many helpful suggestions.

My wife, Ann, has heard many of these ideas so often that she can anticipate my thinking. She has tolerated these unusual interests and research projects in a graceful and supporting way, for which I am grateful.

At Oxford University Press, Peter Ohlin has shepherded this project with professional skill and talent. This is my fifth volume with Oxford. It is a press of great quality for which I express my appreciation.

CONTENTS

LIST OF CASES

Patient, Heal Thyself

The New Medicine

An Introduction

A new medicine is on the horizon. It is as radically different from modern medicine as modern medicine is from medicine men and faith healers. Premodern thinking did not understand scientific notions of cause and effect. It believed in the power of evil spirits, magical forces, and bewitching. It had no understanding of scientific evidence. Modern medicine is nothing if not scientific. At its best it refuses to tolerate, without scientific testing, folk beliefs about causes and cures. It rejects "old wives' tales," deeply held but unproven beliefs about the powers of all manner of strange potions, procedures, and prophecies. Although these more primitive understandings of medicine survive, they come from a paradigm entirely different from the one for the medicine we call modern or scientific.

Modern medicine reached its zenith in the second half of the twentieth century. It was responsible for overpowering infection, generating genetic explanations, and significantly increasing average life expectancy. It was also doomed to its own destruction. It rejected religious and cultural beliefs so radically that it seduced us (both medical scientists and laypeople) into believing that from good science alone we could learn what treatments were "medically appropriate" or "medically indicated." Moderns believed that the physician, at least the ideal physician well-schooled in the science of his or her profession, could determine not only the cause of diseases but also the best treatments for them. They believed that physicians could, based on science, order tests, prescribe drugs, choose surgeries, and even tell laypeople how to make lifestyle choices. Laypeople were told that it was bad for them to smoke and eat fatty foods, good to exercise, bad to be overweight or seriously underweight, and—until recently—bad to consume alcohol. It was as if the facts of science unaided could automatically lead the well-trained, objective medical professional to these "clinical facts." They believed "doctor knows best." We now know none of that is true.

We are headed for a wholesale change—a medicine as different from modern, scientific medicine as the modern practice was from its primitive predecessors. We are in the early stages of what can be called the "new medicine," a medicine in which patients will recapture responsibility for their own health choices—including choosing their own therapies based on their own beliefs and values. It will be a world in which patients will, in a very real sense, have to heal themselves.

It is a medicine that does not reject medical science, but does reject the belief that physicians can ever know what is medically best for their patients based on medical science alone. Although modern medicine believed that medical choices had to be based on science, the new medicine insists that every medical choice requires nonscientific value judgments. It claims that someone's value judgments must be imposed on the scientific facts in order to know what counts as a medically wise choice. Advocates for the new medicine insist that there is no reason that physicians' values should be the ones that are used. In fact, there are good reasons to believe that physicians' values are especially inappropriate ones to use for typical medical decisions. The very experts who have been singled out as the ones who "know best" will turn out to be uniquely poor judges when it comes to the patient's medical interests.

It is not that physicians are incompetent in medical science (although some may be). It is not that physicians are corrupted by their economic self-interest (although some undoubtedly are). Rather, everything said in this book will assume (for purposes of argument) that the vast majority of physicians are reasonably competent in their knowledge of and skills in medicine and are dedicated to their patients' interests rather than their bank accounts. My claim is that this is no longer enough. Physicians no longer can be expected to be able to do what is in their patients' interest just because they are competent physicians. They cannot be expected to do what best serves patients' interests because they cannot be expected to know what patients' interests are. The new medicine will be one that focuses on the value choices that have to be imposed on the facts of medicine in order to decide what is good practice. The new medicine rejects the old slogan, "Doctor knows best."

It will turn to others to make virtually all the critical choices. The conviction of the new medicine is that usually the patient knows best—that is, the patient usually knows the patient's own interests better than the physician or even a whole group of physician professionals.

That won't always be the case. Sometimes—believe it or not—the government or the insurance company may know best. Sometimes parents will; sometimes politicians will. What is unique in what I am calling the new medicine is the insight that only in very special and unusual circumstances will it be the doctor who knows best what is in either the patient's or the community's interest. The new medicine exists in a world in which the doctor's expertise in medical science will have to be combined with the expertise of others—especially the expertise of the patient—in knowing the values upon which literally every decision in medicine must be based.

The result is a medicine that is something totally different from that of the twentieth century. Of course, because the values have to be imposed on good medical science, and physicians for the foreseeable future will be the ones who know the science, this means that we cannot discard the physician. He or she still has an important role, but it is a very different role from the one of modern medicine.

Consider the mess we had gotten ourselves into by the middle of the twentieth century. Modern medicine had produced some dramatic successes. Penicillin—a safe, simple, and cheap drug—easily cured many of the infections that had, until then, been viciously fatal. Injections of insulin preserved lives of people with diabetes. Anesthesia permitted an escape from the agony of surgery and amputations. The choices to use these and countless other miracle treatments seemed so obvious that we tricked ourselves into believing that they could be chosen by competent physicians on the basis of the medical facts alone. It was as if it were a fact that if you had pneumonia, you ought to take penicillin. We failed to see the value judgments because they were so easy and obvious. It is better to live with the very minor risks of penicillin than die without them; it is better to inject the insulin than to suffer the major, sometimes fatal, complications of going without it; it is better to take the remote risks of anesthesia than to suffer the pain without it. Only those with a distorted theology claimed that the suffering was so good for one's character that the pain should be endured. We ceded to physicians the absolute authority to determine when medical interventions were appropriate. We developed the bizarre practice of having physicians prescribe remedies. We believed that somehow the physician was supposed to know which remedies were best for us.

But look where that got us. By the 1960s many states had laws that would permit women to have abortions when and only when a doctor determined they were appropriate—and most physicians almost never did. A mature, college-educated man seeing a physician to diagnose a lump in his abdomen could have the truth of a terminal cancer withheld by the physician because that self-appointed expert had decided that the patient would be better off not knowing. The doctor was permitted to exercise what was called the "therapeutic privilege," that is, the privilege to decide whether the patient would be better off being lied to than knowing the truth. Somehow, we came to believe that knowing the medical facts vested one with the ultimate authority to decide what to do based on those facts. The poor patient was left not only with no choice about whether to have radical surgery, chemotherapy, or radiation, but also with no choices about how to live the remaining days of his of her life.

CASE INTRO. 1

Karen Ann Quinlan: The Groundbreaking Case

The foolishness of the belief that doctor knows best reached the public's consciousness in the United States in 1975. At the time I was the Associate for Medical Ethics at the Institute of Society, Ethics and the Life Sciences—the New York bioethics think tank that has since come to be known at the Hastings Center. I was the staff person in charge of its Research Group on Death and Dying.

I got a telephone call one day from a young lawyer named Paul Armstrong. He was working in a legal aid clinic in New Jersey and had been asked by a couple for help. Their 21-year-old daughter had suffered a terrible accident. After spending some time with friends at a local bar imbibing some alcohol and perhaps also consuming some tranquilizers, she had lost consciousness and stopped breathing. She apparently did not understand the way these two drugs interacted. She ended up unconscious and not breathing. By the time she was rushed to the hospital and given emergency treatment she had suffered such severe brain damage that she would never again regain consciousness.

Paul Armstrong asked me for assistance in helping the parents get her ventilator stopped so she could be allowed to die with whatever dignity could be mustered. I agreed to meet with him and consult in planning legal action.

The young woman, who the world would soon know as Karen Ann Quinlan, had the misfortune of falling into the hands of a physician named Robert Morse, who believed that, as a physician, he could determine what was best for her. I came to call this strange belief the "as a" syndrome—what I considered the first "disease" of the sick phenomenon of modern medicine. He literally had never met her at any point in her life when she was conscious, but he, nevertheless, believed that, as a physician, he could draw on the wisdom of his profession to determine that it was best for her to have life support continue as long as possible. He felt he could reach this judgment in spite of the fact that Karen had reportedly expressed the wish never to be kept alive in such a condition. He reached this conclusion in spite of the fact that her parents, both devout Catholics, knew that their church held that in such cases life support can be considered "extraordinary" and that it was acceptable to withdraw the treatment so that nature could take its course. He reached this conclusion in spite of the fact that Father Trapasso, their family priest, had counseled the family and strongly supported their wish to have the ventilator turned off. Dr. Morse had the arrogance to claim that he was the one to make this decision and that his only obligation was to conform to the standard of practice of his profession—which he claimed was to preserve life as long as possible.

Even in 1975 he was probably wrong about what his colleagues in medicine would do in such a situation. I discussed with Paul Armstrong developing the legal case for Karen's liberation from medical custody by arguing in court that Dr. Morse had made a mistake about the professional consensus. We could argue he was wrong in his view about what his colleagues thought about perpetuating breathing in permanently unconscious patients. I think we could have shown that most physicians would have chosen—even back then—to stop the ventilator.

But that would have implied that the professional consensus of Dr. Morse's colleagues was the proper standard for deciding when life support should cease. It would leave Karen, if not in Dr. Morse's custody, then in the custody of the medical profession. It would cede to this group of strangers the authority to decide when fighting to preserve life is appropriate and when it is not.

This choice simply is not one a physician or a group of physicians ought to have any authority to make. No matter how scientific they were in diagnosing Karen's condition, no matter how accurately they could predict whether she would recover, no matter how wise they were in the science of neurology and the techniques of maintaining respiration in unconscious patients, they were not in any way experts on the value of unconscious life. This was a religious or a philosophical or an ethical decision. When it came to Karen's life, she herself was surely the one who should have had the authority to make that decision insofar as she was able. If she was not, then her parents, as her closest relatives, were the best surrogates. Her friends might be called on to help, and so might her priest. We could even make a case that the broader society should have some say, at least in setting limits on what kinds of patients should be permitted to choose to stop life support. However, Dr. Morse—a person who had no claim to expertise in making these value judgments and knew absolutely nothing about her beliefs and values—seems to be among the least plausible substitutes.

Paul Armstrong, with my encouraging, chose a much bolder and more appropriate course. He argued that, regardless of Dr. Morse's views and the opinion of his professional colleagues, the choice was not his to make. It was Karen's or her family's speaking on her behalf. The New Jersey Supreme Court agreed. In its stilted, formal language, the court spoke the words that would signal the end of modern medicine. It rejected the automatic authority of the standards of the medical profession:

> The question is whether there is such internal consistency and rationality in the application of such standards as should warrant their constituting an ineluctable bar to the effectuation of substantive relief for plaintiff at the hands of the court. We have concluded not.[1]

My students in my graduate seminar on the ethics of death and dying can easily spend 15 minutes deciphering those sentences. The court is trying to decide whether it can use the "standards" of the profession of medicine as the basis for barring the parents' request for a court order that will get the ventilator stopped. The court takes the position that if the professional standards were "internally consistent" and "rational," they might provide a basis for supporting the doctor and refusing to agree with the parents' request. It then concludes that the professional standards fail to provide a basis for barring the parents from taking actions that will get the ventilator stopped.

With that short final sentence, "We have concluded not," the American courts cut patients loose from the tyranny of medical professional authority. That decision and countless others in state and federal courts throughout the land (and eventually throughout the world) started the collapse of the authoritarianism of modern medicine. It signaled that a new medicine was on the horizon, one in which value judgments in medical decisions were seen as inevitable and were presumed to rest with the patient or the agent for the patient rather than the physician.

CASE INTRO. 2

Radical Mastectomy versus Lumpectomy

These life-and-death decisions to forgo life support were not the only examples of modern medicine presuming that the expert on the medical facts was also an expert in making the value judgments. As late as the 1980s patients diagnosed with breast cancer were still being told by their authoritarian oncologists whether a radical mastectomy or a simpler lumpectomy was best for them. Never mind that the science itself was very complex and ambiguous. Medical scientists themselves often were in dispute over whether the radical procedure really increased the chance of preserving life. Never mind that some physicians were insisting on the more radical procedure whereas their colleagues caring for medically identical patients were choosing lumpectomies. The real issue here was that in order to make the decision, one needed to know how important it was to get the psychological satisfaction of feeling like one had done the most aggressive treatment possible. In order to make the decision, one also needed to know how important it was to preserve the appearance and feeling of a normal breast.

It is patently absurd for predominantly male oncologists or surgeons to claim expertise in the really important issues at stake in the choice. It is even offensive for female physicians to claim this authority. Some women, once they are informed about the confused state of the medical science, insist that for them preserving the breast is the critical issue—even if it turns out to produce a somewhat higher risk of mortality. For others the comfort of knowing they have done everything possible is more important than the physical appearance. Surely, no physician can legitimately claim to be an authority on making these value judgments for the patient. The patient, informed about the medical facts, is the one with the critical information. She should be the one to choose among the therapies.

Every Medical Decision Requires Value Judgments

Although the need to introduce the patient's values in Karen Quinlan's case and the mastectomy cases may seem obvious, many might, at this point, consider these exceptions. The choices for abortion, sterilization, forgoing life support, and removing a breast all seem unusually value-laden, and the values seem conspicuous. Nevertheless, even with the increasing prominence of ethically controversial procedures in medicine, if there were nothing more to the convergence of values and medicine, modern medicine could survive as an essentially scientific enterprise. An ever-increasingly large footnote would be necessary to indicate that ethical and other value choices play a special role in these special cases. They would be seen as ethically exotic—unusual in raising serious ethical and other value issues.

The critical problem emerges when we consider more ordinary, routine cases. We need to press further to see if there are medical choices without some kind of value judgments. When I began teaching medical ethics at Columbia University's College of Physicians and Surgeons in 1970, I made an offer to the students. I offered to buy any students a dinner at the best restaurant in town if they could bring me a medical case on their floor that involved absolutely no value judgments. I have renewed the offer from time to time with medical students I teach at Georgetown University, at Albany Medical College's seven-year medical program, and at St. George's University School of Medicine in Grenada.

I have never had to pay off and am quite confident I never will. A quick look at the logical structure of medical decisions convinces the students that they are not going to find such a value-free case. Of course, every medical decision should be based on the facts of medical science, but a decision to perform a test, write a prescription, or give some medical advice always has to go beyond the science. It always has to involve a value judgment about the expected outcome if one course or another is followed.

If clinical decisions are expressed in words, they always have to contain a value term. The physician must say (or assume) something like, "This is the drug that will be good for you," "You ought to have this operation," "This exercise is appropriate for you," or "I advise you to cut down on fatty foods."

Some people might say that when a doctor says something is "appropriate" or "good for you," he or she means it is "medically appropriate or good." However, "medically appropriate or good" turns out not to mean much. All of these terms add something to the medical facts. They evaluate the outcome predicted by medical science if the recommended course is followed and compare it with the consequences of following other courses (including doing nothing at all). They then endorse the outcome that the physician deems most valuable. Sometimes those value judgments are quite obvious. Almost all patients might agree with them. But the fact is that the physician has to make a value judgment. And not every patient will agree. In special cases the patient may totally reject the value judgments. She may be a Christian Scientist who believes that God, rather than the medical professional, heals. He may be at a point in life in which the outcome the physician assumes is good is judged by the patient to be bad. Even death can be considered appropriate by most of us at some point in our lives.

Although most of these inevitable value judgments may be obvious to most people most of the time, when we look more closely at the physician's value choices, we see that some of the choices are not at all obvious. Physicians impose on their patients the choice between a higher dose that runs a slightly greater risk of drowsiness or a lower dose that avoids the drowsiness but may leave the patient with an annoying itch. They choose to give the child an injectable form of a drug, which will supply a more accurate and faster dose, rather than an oral form that will be more comfortable. Meanwhile, some of their colleagues, equally competent but with slightly different values, will make the alternative choices.

We might be inclined to believe that when these value choices must be made, they should be made according to the dominant or majority values of the typical physician. That is what the law calls the "professional standard." It is what Dr. Morse claimed to be using in Karen Quinlan's case. But who is to say that individual patients should have the dominant or average values of the professional group inflicted on them? Actually, good evidence exists that typical physicians impose their value judgments on the medical facts in systematically atypical ways. After all, at least until recently, physicians have been predominantly male, predominantly white, and predominantly wealthy. They have been educated predominantly in the sciences, have been middle-aged or elderly, have had a deep psychological need to work with individuals rather than social or political groups, and generally have ended up on psychological tests as unusually authoritarian. There is even some evidence that they have had unusually traumatic experiences with death at a very early age. It is no wonder that women, children, ethnic minorities, the poor, and the less well educated may think differently and value medical outcomes differently than their physicians.

Patients' Rights: An Alternative to Hippocratic Paternalism

By the 1970s, more aggressive and avant garde laypeople were beginning to resist the imposition of the physician's values on them. We discovered that the old Hippocratic Oath, which physicians were touting as their moral compass, was, in fact, an ethical code of dubious merit.[2] Rather than being an all-purpose, timeless code for good moral practice in medicine, it was increasingly seen for what it was—an initiation oath from a small, pagan, Greek religious cult that extolled a morality that appears closely related to the ideology of the Pythagoreans—the same people that brought us the Pythagorean theorem we learned in geometry.[3] The Pythagoreans were a religious-philosophical-scientific sect with some rather strange moral views. They, like Jews and Christians, opposed abortion and euthanasia—unusual positions in the Greek world at the time. Some believe that this agreement made the Hippocratic Oath appealing so that early Christians accepted this medical ethic rather than one of the other Greek schools of thought. On the other hand, many elements of the Oath are downright offensive to both Jews and Christians. For instance, it was the uniquely elitist Hippocratic view that medical formulas were to be kept secret from patients, reserved only for the initiates. The Oath included a strange prohibition on all surgery, apparently because the Hippocratic cult believed that its members should be kept ritually pure by avoiding contamination with blood. It reflected a militant absence of any sense of a moral community to which physicians might have duties, a view of social responsibility diametrically opposite from Jewish and Christian values. There is nothing in the Oath resembling informed consent. The confidentiality clause is vague and is now rejected by all thinking people. It can be interpreted as permitting physicians to disclose private patient information whenever they think it is in the interest of the patient to do so—even if the patient disagrees. The Oath not only swears by the Greek gods and goddesses, but ends with a prayer that the physician receive fame and glory if he follows the code and the "opposite" if he does not—a view of morality that is heretical to Jews and Christians.[4]

It seems clear to anyone who studies the Oath carefully that a modern physician has a choice. He or she can choose to base medical practice on one of the great religious or secular philosophical systems of the world (such as Christianity or liberal political philosophy) or on the pagan Greek religion of Hippocratism—a strange, antiquated religious/philosophical/ethical system that, by its very nature, excludes all nonphysicians. It raises the question why rational twenty-first century patients would permit physicians to practice medicine on them if those physicians subscribe to this old, morally offensive, elitist, cultic oath.

This insight led to a patients' rights movement in the last decades of the twentieth century. It was undoubtedly a product of the great rights movements of the 1960s, an era that challenged the authority of elites on all fronts. Students and other antiwar activists challenged the authority of military generals to use their personal values to set policy in Vietnam. The civil rights movement challenged the authority of a race to claim superiority. The women's movement challenged the authority of males to dominate. Students challenged the authority of professors and administrators. With civil rights, women's rights, and students' rights, could patients' rights be far behind?

The women's movement produced one of the earliest and most insightful attacks on orthodox modern medicine. Women had had enough of the arrogance of obstetricians condescendingly probing their most personal parts and equally condescendingly deciding how women ought to live. The Boston Women's Health Book Collective produced *Our Bodies, Ourselves,* one of the first militant challenges to modern medicine's view that the one who knows the medical science knows best. Feminist health care is a wonderful, pioneering case of patients with a different worldview properly rejecting the core beliefs of modern medicine.

Even though certain sectarian religious groups held beliefs and values radically different from the feminist health collectives, they also discovered the foolishness of the belief that the one who knows medical science can automatically know what is best for the patient. The Christian Scientists, Seventh Day Adventists, and, especially with regard to blood, the Jehovah's Witnesses all recognized that knowing the facts of medicine gave no guidance on what counted for them as medically appropriate care. Talmudic Jewish medicine and fundamentalist Oral Robert's medical center in Tulsa shared with the militant feminists the crucial insight that one cannot determine what counts as good medicine simply by knowing the facts of medical science. To determine what is good or appropriate medical treatment, one must superimpose some system of beliefs and values—some "ethic"—on the medical facts. For virtually all patients in contemporary times, the Hippocratic ethic is not the right choice.

Most competent physicians have, by now, wisely abandoned Hippocratism in favor of some other, more plausible belief system. Nevertheless, these physicians will still hold beliefs and values that they will subtly impose on their patients. The value system being imposed on the patient may be no more appropriate for the patient than the old Hippocratic one. For the new medicine, it is not enough for the medical profession to clean up its code of ethics, replacing the most offensive parts of the Hippocratic Oath with some newer views of the group's members. The new medicine is one that combines the knowledge of modern medical science with a recognition that every medical choice must use someone's beliefs and values in deciding what is appropriate. It rejects the suggestion that it is the physician's beliefs and values that should be used—even if they have been modernized. It gives priority to the patient's own beliefs and values. Normally the patient will have to be the primary decision maker in the new medicine.

In its more sophisticated form, the new medicine recognizes that some patients will have to rely on surrogates—parents, guardians, and designated agents—to make some of the value choices on the patient's behalf. It recognizes that for some medical value choices, the course chosen can have such radical impact on others in society that the values of those affected (or the values of the society as a whole) must be considered in order to place limits on individual patient choices. Some drug uses are just too dangerous to the interests of others. Speed (methamphetamine), perhaps heroin and marijuana, and definitely alcohol are drugs that are too dangerous to leave completely to the discretion of individuals. But even in these cases there is no rational reason why the physician's personal beliefs and values will be relevant in deciding whether the patient should have access. The physician may have views about whether a narcotic for a patient in severe pain is worth the risk—to the patient and to the society—but that physician's views cannot be definitive in deciding whether to take that risk. If the patient doesn't want to take the risk, that should settle the matter. He should have the right to endure his pain. But even if the patient is willing to take such a risk, society will need to have a voice, at least when the risks at stake include those to other people. What is critical is that the physician's opinion about whether these risks are worth it just doesn't count in any special way. Having a physician choose whether to write a prescription for a narcotic makes no sense.

The Terminology: Consumer, Customer, or Client–Patient, Partner, or Person

If the new medicine will radically transform the role of the patient into the dominant or primary decision maker, leaving the physician in a much more derivative or secondary role, it is probably time to ask whether the word we use for the beneficiary of the physician's concern has outlived its usefulness. *Patient* is, after all, a provocative term. It comes from the same Latin root that conveys passivity and suffering (as in "long-suffering one willing to tolerate whatever burdens are imposed"). From the standpoint of one trying to reclaim a proper role as autonomous medical decision maker responsible for his or her own medical fate, patient is an odd term to preserve. In the new medicine patients can be patient no longer.

That being said, it is a complex and controversial task to come up with a replacement term. One branch of the patients' rights movement has substituted the word *consumer*. Drawing on libertarian, free-market principles, the layperson interacting with the health professional is considered a consumer in the market sense of the term. Some even more committed to the market model have used the term *customer*. But seeing the layperson as mere consumer or customer is not much better when it comes to challenging the passive image of the term *patient*. To be one who merely consumes medical knowledge and services does not go far in placing the patient in charge. To think of the layperson as a customer is far too mercantile a metaphor.

The nursing profession deserves credit for sensing the offensiveness of the term *patient*. Early on in the evolution from modern to postmodern health care, the American Nurses Association started referring to the layperson with whom nurses were interacting as the client. *Client* has a more professional sound to it than does *consumer*. It is what lawyers call their counterparts. Being a client seems to convey more dignity than being a consumer. It even implies that the layperson has something of a voice in decision making. But *client* is still a subordinating term. Vassal states totally dependent on some superpower are called "client" states. The term *client* also implies passivity. It derives from the Latin *cleans*, which simply means "dependent."

By 1970, the year that might appropriately mark the beginning of the transition to the new era in medicine and medical ethics, the senior statesman of the field, Paul Ramsey, put forward the radical idea that the patient should be thought of simply as a person.[5] Ramsey, the Methodist theologian and chair of the Religion Department at Princeton, spent two academic semesters on the floors of Georgetown University Hospital developing a new understanding of the links between ethics and medicine. His association with Catholic obstetrician Andre Hellegers led to the founding of the Kennedy Institute of Ethics, the bioethics research institute where I have spent the last three decades of my life. Ramsey understood the patient/physician relation as one of fidelity—faithfulness of each party to the other grounded in a common set of beliefs and values. For him, each of the participants must be thought of as persons in the fullest, most noble sense of the term. Each is responsible for the decisions he or she makes. Those decisions have to be grounded in a broad belief system, which, for Ramsey, was the Christian tradition. This belief system extends far beyond medicine and shapes one's very understanding of what medicine is about. It would, for him, be impossible to understand what medicine required without embedding medicine deeply within a fundamental belief system, a system that not only conveyed the meaning and end of life, but also specified the moral framework for pursuing those ends. He was satisfied only when the patient was reconceptualized as a whole person, an active, responsible member of a moral community.

During the 1970s, I was an enthusiastic supporter of Paul Ramsey, as well as a militant critic. Ramsey was a member of the Hastings Center's Research Group on Death and Dying, the group that I was administering when I was asked to assist in the liberation of Karen Quinlan from her medical captors. I agreed with most of what Ramsey said about patients needing to be thought of as whole persons actively responsible for their health care, but I took more seriously than Ramsey the plurality of worldviews— religious and secular—upon which one might realistically base medical choices. Although I continue to share much of Ramsey's theological and philosophical framework for my own personal medical decisions, I also recognize that there are many other worldviews out there upon which others will make their choices. In fact, there are as many systems for making medical choices as there are religious and philosophical beliefs in the world. Although Ramsey was content to articulate his conservative Protestant beliefs about what was the correct basis for making medical choices, I take even more seriously than he the limits of human finitude. I am less sure I have the right set of religious and philosophical beliefs to impose on others. I am even less sure I can persuade the rest of the world that the ones I have chosen are the right ones. I am thus more content to assume that for the foreseeable future in the postmodern world, we will have no agreement on the definitively correct set of beliefs and values. That will mean there will continue to be many "medicines," as many as there are systems of belief and value. Every physician will have to be seen as practicing medicine according to one of those systems of belief and value, and every patient will have to be seen as making his or her medical choices on the basis of one of them. This means that, for me, the postmodern world of the new medicine must rely on the pairing up of physicians and patients according to compatible belief systems about what the ends or purposes of medicine ought to be. This has led me to focus on the patient as one of the partners in the lay-professional relation. I even once wrote a pair of books on research and clinical medical ethics entitled *The Patient as Partner*. The patient will be increasingly the dominant or primary partner (the "managing partner," to use a corporate metaphor), the one whose beliefs and values must dominate. Nevertheless, the health professional—the nurse, pharmacist, dentist, and other health professionals, as well as the physician—will also be a partner in the process. Health professionals will inevitably draw on their personal beliefs and values in shaping communications and choosing which facts and which treatment options to present to the layperson. Health professionals will, in this sense, be the secondary decision makers, the secondary partners in the relation, but nevertheless ones with responsibilities as well as rights.

In the end, none of these terms—*consumer* or *customer, client; patient, person*, or *partner*—adequately does the whole job we are seeking in a term for the layperson in the new medicine. I have considered insisting that we completely abandon the term *patient*, both because of its offensive root meaning and its offensive association with the old role in modern, authoritarian Hippocratic medicine, but I end by concluding that the term will probably not go away. In new medicine we will instead have to reconstruct the term to add to it a new dignity, a new authority, and a new activism. In that sense, the new patient will have elements of all of the other terms. He or she will be part consumer, part client, part customer, but especially a whole person who is the senior partner in the relation with health professionals acting as assistants.

This new medicine is based on the primacy of the patient and the logical necessity of value choices in every move made in the medical partnership between patient and professional provider. That simple notion will require abandoning the way we think and talk about virtually every aspect of medical care. It will require adopting a radically new vocabulary and mindset. This book sets out the far-reaching implications.

In part I, I explore some typical cases that show how this new medicine requires thinking that is different from that of modern medicine. Then, starting with chapter 4 and continuing through chapters 5 and 6, I provide a fuller account of why the doctor no longer can be presumed to know what is best for the patient. Chapters 7, 8, and 9 show why the old language of modern medicine—terms like "doctors orders," "medically indicated treatment," and being "discharged" from the hospital—can no longer be used. Notions of "medically necessary treatment" and "treatment of choice, " so important in deciding what health insurance will cover, are unmasked as code words for someone's value judgments.

Part II introduces some new concepts and terms—notions that will replace consent (chapters 10 and 11) and prescription writing (chapter 12). Once the legitimacy of the practice of prescription writing is challenged, it will have to be replaced with some new approach to the use of medications.

An alternative to prescriptions will be presented in chapter 13. In chapters 14 and 15 I will rethink our concept of obesity and the role of the physician in weight management. I will ask the deceptively tricky question, "Are fat people overweight?" Chapter 16 explores the implications of a new understanding of medicine for health insurance and, in particular, the idea that a fair insurance system would provide the same coverage for everyone. In chapter 17 I argue that morally just health insurance would require that different people get different lists of covered services. We shall also see that some more innovative and attractive forms of medical care, such as the hospice for the terminally ill, will have to be reconceptualized (chapter 18). In chapter 19 I will argue that hospice should not be part of health insurance in the new medicine.

Part III turns to the way the new medicine will think about broader social aspects of health care including recruiting subjects into research (chapters 20 and 21), clinical practice guidelines and treatment protocols (chapter 22), outcomes research (chapter 23), and using the consensus of experts to establish medical facts (chapter 24). The volume closes with a "Patient Manifesto," a succinct summary of what patients will demand in their new role as the primary decision makers in the new medicine—one in which they will make healing decisions for themselves.

The writer of the biblical proverb was tough on physicians when he offered the often-quoted demand, "Physician, heal thyself." I am easier on the medical professional. I am, after all, assuming that he or she is reasonably competent and dedicated to their patients' welfare. But in another way, I am more radical. I claim that the very fabric of medicine must be reconceptualized. Doctors—even competent and dedicated ones—will no longer be seen as capable of determining what will benefit their patients. It is patients themselves who, in the world of the new medicine, have to take charge. They will have to be the ones choosing the beliefs and values upon which health-care interventions must be based. In this sense, my imperative goes beyond the biblical author's. It pleads, "Patient, heal thyself."

I

WHY DOCTOR DOES NOT KNOW BEST

ONE The Puzzling Case of the Broken Arm

This book rests on the claim that every medical decision requires value judgments that cannot be based on science. It would not be surprising if this claim were greeted with some healthy skepticism. Almost anyone would grant that some medical decisions are heavily shaped by religious and other values. Abortion, euthanasia, and even organ transplants raise profound moral and philosophical questions about the meaning and value of life. No doctor, however good a practitioner, can decide whether an abortion is "medically indicated" because the decision is always an evaluative one. Even in the increasingly rare case of a woman's life being jeopardized by a pregnancy, science alone cannot tell whether the abortion should occur.

I have counseled patients and physicians having to choose whether to continue an all-out battle against death, even at the expense of a terribly painful, disfiguring surgery. For one man, life was so precious that he left no doubt that for him, the battle should proceed. He was willing to undergo a hemicorpectomy (the amputation of his entire body below the waist) for a chance to live. On the other hand, I have counseled a young woman facing a heart transplant, for whom the perpetual agony of antirejection medication and fear of relapse was so overwhelming that for her, the transplant was not the right choice. She wanted to refuse, even though it meant a certain early death.

By the end of the twentieth century some physicians and almost all patients recognized these decisions as "ethically loaded" value choices that
physicians had to cede to their patients. There is, however, a new medicine
emerging. The new medicine pushes much further. It claims that not only
these ethically dramatic cases but literally every medical choice—no matter
how mundane—inevitably requires value judgments and that physicians
make them only by imposing their personal and often idiosyncratic views
on their patients. Their equally competent colleagues facing similar choices
but holding slightly different values would choose differently, even though
they agreed completely about the medical facts.

If you are skeptical, in the remainder of this chapter and in the one that
follows consider three real cases I have encountered. I choose these precisely
because they seem so routine and trivial that many would be tempted to
claim they are devoid of value judgments. Names and details are changed to
provide anonymity, but the stories are described as they happened.

CASE I.I

The Puzzling Case of the Broken Arm

Phil was a sophomore in his state's premier university in a city some
hundred miles from his home. Playing "severe Frisbee" one fall afternoon, he dove for the disc and landed on his right wrist. He knew in-
stantly it was broken. His buddies drove him to the school clinic,
where the arm was set. In a few weeks he was as good as new—almost.

The arm was left with a slight distortion that concerned the
orthopedist but did not appear to require surgical correction. The
next summer when Phil was skating at a roller rink with his friends,
he fell on the arm and rebroke it. This time the orthopedic surgeon
said pins would have to be placed to reconstruct the bone. The surgery was uneventful. The surgeon instructed Phil and his parents
that he would have to return for removal of the pins in about a year
when the bone was mended.

The following summer the procedure was scheduled for Phil as an
outpatient. Everything went fine. His now-screwless arm was placed
once again in a cast so the screw holes could mend.

In the conversation with Phil and his parents after the successful
events, the surgeon made a statement that was rather remarkable,
even though neither he nor Phil at first realized all its implications.

He said, "Most surgeons would leave this cast on for about seven weeks, but I found that if you are careful, I can remove it in about four weeks, so schedule an appointment in a month and we'll get it off."

Phil and his parents here encounter an amazing array of value judgments made by the surgeon. Pass over all the judgments not to place the pins after the first break and to place them after the second. Forget about the techniques used in setting the arm each time, the type of surgery, the anesthesia, the decision to remove the pins after a year. There is no reason to doubt that each of these decisions easily conformed to the practices of orthopedic surgeons. Of course, they all involved value judgments, but they were judgments that would probably lead to little controversy. Let's focus on the decision about when the cast should be removed.

First, this surgeon says something very controversial. He announces to his patient what the standard practice is for removing the cast: His colleagues generally removed it after seven weeks. He then tells Phil and his parents that he was going to depart from the standard practice—an announcement that surely would have alarmed the surgeon's lawyer had he heard it. Practitioners of modern medicine might be concerned as well. Modern medicine assumes that there is a correct number of weeks to leave a cast on in these circumstances and that a consensus among orthopedists is good (if not perfect) evidence of how many weeks that is. In the days of modern medicine, Phil would have been left wondering why he should go with his surgeon's four-week plan rather than the consensus seven. Some might even say that the surgeon has not only made a mistake, but foolishly announced the error to the patient.

The new medicine sees the situation very differently. Phil's surgeon doesn't actually give Phil a clear reason for this deviation, but we can perhaps deduce it. He says that if Phil is careful, he can have the cast removed three weeks earlier. It appears that the surgeon assumes that wearing a cast is an unpleasant experience, so removing it early is a good thing. Likewise, one might guess that the surgeon believes it is not a terribly onerous task to be careful.

It now becomes clear that there is no objectively correct number of weeks to leave the cast on the arm for this kind of surgery. The more cast-averse one is and the more comfortable one is trying to be careful, the earlier the cast should come off. On the other hand, for those who live an active life, are nervous about having to try to avoid the risk of injury of the unprotected arm, and are not particularly troubled by the cast, a longer period is surely the right answer.

Now, of course, there are some periods so short that almost no one would find the time adequate. The risk of reinjury and the nuisance of being careful enough would be overwhelming. On the other hand, there would be some lengths of time so long that almost no one would see them as necessary. The extra value of going beyond the standard seven weeks would add so little protection that only the most compulsive would be attracted. In fact, if the cast were left on long enough, the disutilities of muscle atrophy would be another reason to get the cast removed.

Something as utterly trivial and devoid of moral controversy as when to remove a cast turns out to depend on the value trade-offs of the one making the choice. Phil's surgeon is not making a clear-cut mistake when he deviates from the standard of practice. If the surgeon is really averse to the cast and really uncomfortable with one on his arm, then he is rationally inclined to get it off earlier. For him, four weeks may be just the right time (even though his colleagues have made the value trade-off in a way that leads to the seven-week period). It is not irrational for the surgeon to favor a shorter time for removing the cast, even if he knows his colleagues choose seven weeks and even if he agrees completely with them on all of the relevant facts.

The problem, however, is that it is not the surgeon's arm that is in the cast. It's Phil's. Discovering that the decision about when to remove a cast is a value judgment takes it away from the consensus standard of practice of the surgeon's colleagues, but, logically, it also takes it away from the surgeon. If a value trade-off must be made between the nuisance of the cast and the nuisance of being careful without it, it should be Phil's values that get traded off, not those of his surgeon or those of surgeons in general.

If this is right, then we reach a remarkable conclusion: Neither Phil's surgeon nor the community of competent orthopedic surgeons can know when is the right time to remove Phil's cast. In fact, we can no longer talk about any such thing as an all-purpose, generic correct time.

Phil ends up surprising his surgeon. He points out that he would be returning to school soon. It will be a two-hour trip each way to come back in four weeks to get the cast removed. He realizes, however, that in five weeks his school will have a break. He will be home for the break, so he can easily come to get the cast removed without missing class. For him, five weeks is the right length of time for cast to be on his arm, and it had nothing to do with the orthopedic issues.

| Hernias, Diets, and Drugs

Another case similarly shows how the value judgments made by physicians permeate every move made by practitioners, even when neither they nor their patients perceive it.

CASE 2.1

Driving after Hernia Repair

Mr. Westin had noticed a protruding lump in his lower abdomen and a nagging pain in his groin area. He asked his HMO internist about it during a physical exam. The internist suspected a hernia and referred Mr. Westin to the HMO's surgery department. The surgeon concurred. He indicated there was no urgency, but that the hernia should be repaired surgically sometime in the next year or so.

Mr. Westin had planned a vacation that was a dream of a lifetime, a six-month trip to Asia, Australia, and New Zealand. He was scheduled to leave in eight months. He decided to put off the surgery until after he returned.

The trip was a huge success, as was the same-day surgery after he returned. His surgeon said to him afterward, "You can ride in a car right away, but don't drive for a week." Mr. Westin wondered how the surgeon knew that was the correct recommendation.

Once again, we see a very routine medical exchange without any unexpected complications or controversy. Still, the value judgments come early and often, even if the players don't recognize them. When Mr. Westin is worried enough about the lump and the discomfort, he makes a value judgment to seek some advice. He chooses not to turn to a religious healer, to pray, or to consult a health food store clerk, but to raise the concern with his HMO internist. The internist decides to spend the HMO's resources by referring him to a surgeon who thinks it is not an urgent problem, but one that eventually should be corrected. Mr. Westin could decide he doesn't want to worry about the hernia during his trip and so ask for the operation before he departs, but instead he reflects a set of values in which, on balance, he prefers doing the surgery later—risking that the hernia might require more urgent attention while he is traveling.

All of these are value judgments. Different physicians and patients with different values would make them differently. But let's focus on the last value judgment and ask whether the surgeon has a basis for telling Mr. Westin that he can ride in the car but not drive for week.

The surgeon's underlying concern is that stress on the surgical wound could cause it to open and interfere with the healing. The conservative course would be to strive to minimize that stress. The fact that the surgeon does not object to riding in the car shows he is not as conservative as he could be. Driving, however, involves somewhat more stress on the wound—controlling the gas and brake. The most intriguing question is how the surgeon knows that a week is the right amount of time to ride without driving.

This is a rather subtle set of judgments. Presumably, the surgeon needs an estimate of the different stress on the wound from riding and driving and needs to understand the difference in wound injury rates on day six and day eight. Moreover, even assuming the surgeon has an accurate knowledge of these risk rates, he also needs to know how much risk is worth taking. Most critically, however, he needs to know how important it is for Mr. Westin to drive.

If Mr. Westin is a single parent of modest means and has no way to get his children to school without driving, he is in a very different position from someone who is one of two parents in a family or someone who is sufficiently rich to have a chauffeur and who drives only for recreation. In telling Mr. Westin not to drive for a week, the physician has to consider not only the appropriate risks for him to take, but also what would happen to him if he didn't drive. It seems unlikely that the surgeon had any basis for making these value judgments. This next case is one I discuss with medical students and have included in a case book I and some colleagues have published.[1] It requires the same conclusion.

CASE 2.2

Exercise, Diet, or Drugs to Lower Cholesterol

Jake knew he had a problem. He was 37 years old. At 5′10″ and 220 pounds, he was heavier than his doctor would have liked. His sedentary lifestyle as an information technology specialist at a major accounting firm meant he didn't get the exercise that his wife and his physician thought he should get. His physical exams over the past several years showed a nagging increase in total cholesterol levels (237 mg/dl), and the bad stuff was too high, the good too low. His physician had twice recommended that he exercise at least three days a week and modify his diet to lower the cholesterol. Jake went partway. He cut down on eggs for breakfast. He didn't like them much anyway. He intentionally signed up for the cheaper parking lot at work, which forced him to walk about three blocks to his office. He knew, however, that this wasn't exactly what his physician had in mind.

Now at a routine trip to his HMO, his doctor got on Jake's case again about diet and exercise. The physician continued to worry about the cholesterol. He pointed out that the treatment protocol at the HMO indicated that diet and exercise should bring the cholesterol down to an acceptable level, but if they didn't, Jake was going to have to go on one of the new cholesterol-lowering medications called statins.

The effect on Jake was not what the physician had expected. A question occurred to Jake. He thought to himself, "Do you mean I could get the same cholesterol reduction by simply taking the pill and still eat what I have been eating and not changing my diet or signing up for the plan at the local gym?" Jake considered his options: (1) ask the doctor to put him on a statin now, (2) intentionally avoid the diet and exercise regimen until his next physical exam, when the physician would discover that his cholesterol was still too high and, on his own, would write the prescription for the statins, or

(3) attempt to follow more faithfully the physician's recommendation about diet and exercise to see if the cholesterol problem will be taken care of. Of course, there was a fourth option—take his chances and continue with the high cholesterol unmedicated and uncontrolled by either diet or exercise.

Jake is, undoubtedly, not the only one presented with these choices. In the era of modern medicine, the patient who is told he has high cholesterol and that he should increase exercise and change his diet meekly assumed the physician was right. He might not have liked what he heard. He might not have mustered the willpower to follow the recommendation. But he would have felt guilty if he didn't. He would have assumed that the physician had it right—that the cholesterol needed to be lowered and that diet and exercise are the first course to be tried. In fact, even the current direct-to-consumer television advertising of the statin drugs for lowering cholesterol repeats the wisdom that the drugs should be reserved for cases in which diet and exercise have not done the job.

But in the world of postmodern medicine, Jake may have to probe a little deeper. He might ask how it is that his physician (or the medical profession as a whole) can know that the cholesterol has to be lowered and that the first, best course is diet and exercise. When one thinks about it, it is remarkable that script writers for the television commercials (or their health professional informants) can know exactly when cholesterol levels are too high and that, when they are, diet and exercise are the first treatment of choice. How can they know that for Jake—whom they have never met—this is the right course? How can even his HMO physician know that?

The first problem is figuring out at exactly what level one's cholesterol is too high. It might seem that the answer is obvious—whenever a lower level would lead to the expectation of a longer life or a life with fewer medical problems. But even that presumed standard poses a problem. It probably will turn out that the cholesterol level at which medical problems first begin to show up is not exactly the same as the level at which mortality risk first begins to increase. Moreover, it is unlikely either of these levels is exactly the same for each person. So knowing the level that signals health risks is a more complex problem than we might think.

More critically, how does Jake's physician (or the medical community in general) know that the slightest upturn in mortality or morbidity risk justifies efforts to lower cholesterol? Most data about risks show a pattern. As a risk factor like cholesterol increases, the risk at first begins to rise ever so slowly. It then rises very gradually until eventually the risk is dramatic.

But at no point along the way is there a dramatic jump from an acceptable risk to an unacceptable one.

Consider, for example, speeding in an automobile. If we assume that speed limits are set at some adequately safe level, going one mile per hour faster would seem to be only a tiny bit more dangerous. The increased risk is so small that it is probably impossible to measure without extremely large samples. Adding another mile per hour above the speed limit must add another negligible amount of extra risk. The increase for the second mile is probably just slightly larger than the increase for the first mile, but neither of those extra miles will add more than a tiny amount of extra risk. One can add several one-mile increments one at a time and still get only an imperceptible increase in risk.

In fact, the same is true in reverse about miles below the speed limit. It is not that one is exactly as safe if everyone were going 55 miles per hour on an open highway as one would be if everyone were going 50. Everyone going 50 must be slightly safer. Our society has, however, in its collective wisdom, determined that the risk at 55 miles per hour, even though it is a bit greater than at 50, is low enough that 55 is a reasonable limit. Those wise citizens, however, have determined that going above 55, even though the difference at 56 is only imperceptibly greater, is too great. Of course, some individual citizens make their own risk/benefit calculations and conclude that, for them, 56 is safe enough (even factoring in the extra risk that could come from getting a speeding ticket). In fact, some people calculate that 60 or 65 is safe enough. Depending on what they need to do with the extra seconds they save, how much they worry about the extra risk of the accident, and how much they are troubled by intentional violation of the law, they will discover that, for them, the proper speed to drive on the highway may not be exactly 55. I followed a lady recently who must have calculated that 35 was her ideal. The 55-mile-an-hour limit is, at best, an approximation of what is the wisest speed for the average driver with average skills and average need to get some place quickly.

As more and more miles are added above the speed limit, the risk increases faster and faster. By the time one is 30 or 40 miles an hour over the speed limit, it is obvious there is a serious risk, but at no point is it easy to determine exactly when the risk becomes too great. The pattern is what scientists call a *growth curve*. Figure 2.1 shows what they look like.

A similar problem exists with the cholesterol data. If a physician says total cholesterol should be below 200 mg/dl, she is saying that at that point the risk is going up and at such a rate that, in her opinion, it is not worth it. The problem for the new medicine is how she can know that for this

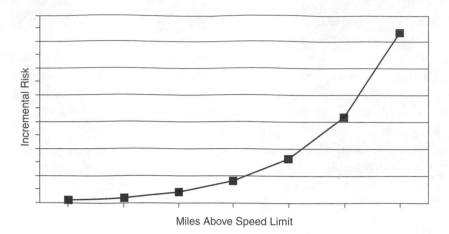

FIGURE 2.1. A Typical Growth Curve.

patient—with his unique beliefs, values, tastes, and desires—the tiny increase in risk from, say, 200 mg to 210 mg is a risk that is not worth taking. At best she can say that by the time Jake reaches 237 mg, the risk is
obviously too great. He is driving at 85 miles per hour. In effect, the physician must say to herself that even though she really doesn't know much
about Jake's life—his desire for high-cholesterol foods, his repulsion for exercise, or his preference to program computers rather than run on tread-
mills—she can know that getting Jake's cholesterol below 200 mg is good
for Jake. Moreover, she seems to know that based on Jake's idiosyncratic
values and preferences, 200 mg is low enough and it is not worth it to try
to get Jake's cholesterol down to 180 (or 160).

From the perspective of the new medicine, these are things Jake's doctor
cannot know. It is simply impossible for Jake's physician to know enough to
determine that Jake should get his cholesterol down to 200 (but that he
need not worry about getting it any lower than 200).

Assume that somehow Jake's doctor solves this problem. She receives a
revelation that 200 mg/dl is the right number for Jake. In order to urge
diet and exercise as the first, best strategy before medication is tried, she
has to know even more about Jake. Presumably, the insight behind the
common wisdom that diet and exercise should be tried first rests on the
awareness that all drugs that can effectively lower cholesterol have some
side effects. They can cause liver damage or a breakdown of muscle tissue.
They can also cause fatigue. The common advice to try diet and exercise
first is based on the belief that they do not have such side effects and that it

is better, therefore, to try them first. It is as if it were a fact that diet and exercise are better than drugs with side effects.

That, of course, is silly. Both diet and exercise *do* have side effects. Any exercise one can imagine poses some risks. Often they seem trivial, but they can include blisters, stress fractures, and being hit by cars while jogging. More critically, for some people exercise is excruciatingly unpleasant. For every runner's high, there are many very low, lows. Deciding whether the exercise is worth it even if it lowers cholesterol is not an easy calculation.

The same can be said for diet. It turns out that the relation of diet to cholesterol is complicated. Much of the body's cholesterol is manufactured internally; it doesn't come from the diet at all. But even if it did, the real question is whether the benefit of the low-cholesterol diet is worth it. That will depend on how much pleasure one gets from high-cholesterol foods and how miserable one is eating sticks, grasses, and other wholesome alternatives.

There is even a more subtle, cultural variable at stake here. Some people, in defense of diet and exercise, may claim that diet and exercise are at least natural lifestyle remedies whereas the drugs are dangerous, toxic chemicals. There exists today a widely held, romantic view that natural treatments and lifestyle changes are preferable. They are believed to be safer, purer, or more virtuous. That, of course, is nothing more than nonscientific beliefs, values, and preferences escalated to the level of cultural value orientation.

Humans are known to have very basic orientations to their lives and culture.[2] Some are optimists, others pessimists; some are doers, others dreamers; some believe in the good in their fellow humans, others in the evil; some believe that in the end, natural, nonmedical interventions are better and safer than pharmacological and other medical ones.

I recently told my wife that a medication I was taking was an old medicine that originally was extracted from a plant. Her first response was, "Oh, it is probably safer." My equally uninformed instinct was, "If it is an old 'natural' botanical, it must be more risky." It does not have the benefit of being designed in a laboratory with the intention of incorporating all the good features of a chemical molecule while engineering all the bad features out. Some of us instinctually think that things growing in nature are safer, purer, or otherwise better.[3] We don't have faith in human chemical engineering. Others are more optimistic about human abilities to improve on nature. Some of us prefer drugs to fix our problems; some prefer behaviors perceived as "natural" such as diet and exercise. Neither approach is necessarily better in the end. Some old "botanicals" derived from plants can be very dangerous. Some are harmless or even healthy. The same is true for synthetic chemicals.

Diet and exercise involve chemicals just as drugs do. In fact, all foods are made up of nothing more than chemicals. Exercise produces chemical changes in the body as well. It is a "faith statement" to affirm a belief in one kind of chemicals rather than the other. Those who believe in natural lifestyle interventions over drugs have every right to their beliefs. But they are beliefs nonetheless. If a patient chooses diet and exercise because she believes them to be better or purer or more holy, she has every right to do so. If the physician imposes those beliefs on a patient who does not share these basic value orientations, she is imposing her own cultural beliefs and values, not practicing scientific medicine.

In order to treat as a fact the claim that diet and exercise are the first, best treatment for high cholesterol, it must be a fact that the risks, harms, and displeasure of the diet and exercise are less than those of the drug that produces a similar lowering of cholesterol. For some people they probably are, and if they have high cholesterol and want to lower it, they should try diet and exercise first. For others the disutilities of diet and exercise may be great enough and those of drugs trivial enough that the statins are really the first, best treatment, assuming that the patient is not better off simply toughing it out with the somewhat elevated cholesterol. (His life may be shorter but happier because of it.)

In the era of modern medicine, determining when one's cholesterol was too high and what to do about it was a matter of medical fact. One could rely on one's doctor to do the blood tests, check the charts, and prescribe—first diet and exercise, and then drugs. In the era of the new medicine, Jake's cholesterol may still be too high, but it is going to be very difficult—almost impossible—for his doctor to know this without a long, complicated conversation with Jake to find out about his beliefs, values, and preferences about diet, exercise, drugs, and quality and length of life.

In the next four chapters, I want to back away from these case examples—the broken arm, the hernia, and the patient with high cholesterol—and outline a more general, theoretical understanding of why the doctor cannot know what is best for his or her patients. In the process I will show that doctors often must stop trying to make decisions that benefit patients.

THREE

Why Physicians Cannot Know What Will Benefit Patients

With these case examples of how value judgments penetrate even the most seemingly routine medical decisions, it is time to step back and look at the problem more systematically. This chapter sets out the core issue—the doctor cannot be expected to know what is best for his or her patients. Then in the next three chapters I will show some reasons why sometimes patient benefit has to be sacrificed to protect patient rights, why sometimes it has to yield to societal interests, and then set out a new limited role for twenty-first-century physicians.

The essence of traditional, that is, "modern," medical ethics can be summed up with the slogan, "The physician should always do what is best for the patient" or, put in the vernacular, "Doctor knows best." That is the core of the Hippocratic Oath in which the physician pledges to work "for the benefit of the sick according to my ability and judgment."[1] It was reflected in the American Medical Association's principles at the beginning of the twentieth century in the injunction "Physicians should not only be ever ready to obey the calls of the sick and the injured, but should be mindful of the high character of their mission and of the responsibilities they must incur in the discharge of momentous duties."[2]

Medical ethics entered the twentieth century with this patient-benefiting focus pretty much intact. It entered the twenty-first with the Hippocratic slogan in a shambles. By the end of the current century, I expect the Hippocratic ethic will be relegated to the ash heap of history—dismissed as a benevolently paternalistic morality that may have worked for a culture in which patients were patient—when they were (as the word *patient* implies) passive, long-suffering, ignorant, and believed to be incapable of making choices—but makes no sense in a complex culture in which patients and their health providers often live in different worlds.

Despite the near-universal reciting of the "patient-benefit" platitude, it is becoming increasingly clear that no one really believes that physicians should literally always try to do everything that they think will benefit their patients. Or at least no one would believe this who really understood the implications. Quite a number of patients would have their interests served best if their personal physician stayed with them in their homes 24 hours a day, yet no one ever advocates that they do so. No one who understands all that would be required to gain a knowledge of what is best for a patient believes that the physician can even know this information. That would require knowledge of the patient's beliefs, values, preferences, cultural commitments, and idiosyncratic inclinations—more than we have a right to expect from even the most dedicated physician. The time has come to debunk the platitude, slaughter the slogan. I expect that debunking to be the story of medical ethics over the next century, the foundation of the new medical ethic.

There are three ways in which I expect the Hippocratic ethic to be challenged:

1. Physicians will discover that they cannot be expected to know what will benefit their patients, which will be the theme of this chapter.
2. Even if physicians know what will benefit their patients, they will be constrained from benefiting in order to fulfill some fundamental moral duties to patients. I'll make this case in the next chapter.
3. At times benefiting patients will so jeopardize the interests or the rights of third parties that physicians will be morally and legally prohibited from providing the benefits. That is the argument of the following chapter.

The result is three reasons why physicians will be forced to abandon their traditional Hippocratic commitment to benefit patients. Then in chapter 6 I will suggest a limited, more realistic way in which physicians in the future will be able to continue their commitment to patient well-being by serving as their advocates or assistants in the medical realm.

The first problem that we discovered with the Hippocratic patient-benefiting ethic in the twentieth century is that it is very hard—indeed usually impossible—for physicians to know what actions on their part will truly benefit their patients. We began that century (and many people have ended it) still believing that "doctor knows best," that is, that somehow a physician could be expected—at least in the ideal case—to be able to know what actions would be beneficial to patients.

In the old Hippocratic cult of ancient Greece knowledge was considered esoteric, potent, and dangerous in the hands of those not initiated into the cult. The cult's members believed that knowledge had to stay in the hands of the elite. Moreover, given that it was a homogeneous culture, there was little disagreement about what would count as a beneficial outcome. The all-knowing initiate into Hippocratic wisdom merely had to decide what would be beneficial based on his judgment (practitioners were exclusively male) and then prescribe.

In the last third of the twentieth century, however, that view collapsed. We now know that even in the ideal case, physicians generally have no basis for knowing what would benefit their patients. Even if they can accurately diagnose disease and predict its future course under various treatment options, they still cannot be expected to have any basis for knowing that one outcome is better than another for the patient who presents the medical problem to them. There are at least three parts to the problem: (1) separating medical and total well-being, (2) distinguishing different kinds of medical well-being, and (3) choosing how to balance benefits and harms.

Why Physicians Cannot Know a Patient's Best Interests: Total Well-Being versus Medical Well-Being

The first part of the problem is that during the last decades of the twentieth century we gained much greater insight into the complex relationship between medical goods and other legitimate goods on a patient's agenda. In contrast to early Hippocratic or early Judeo-Christian times, we now have a considerable division of labor when it comes to "the good" for a person. In early times there was no sharp differentiation between medical goods and other goods such as the psychological, economic, spiritual, aesthetic, legal, familial, or social. The same all-purpose wise man was expected to give advice in any of these areas. Medical matters were integrated with the other spheres. Disease, for example, was seen as punishment from God for wrongful behavior.

By the beginning of the twenty-first century, we still have not completely sorted out these relationships. For example, there remains considerable confusion over the links between the organic and the psychological. We still do not know whether schizophrenia is dependent on some genetic, organic cause or on psychological and familial interactions. Undoubtedly, both play some role. We still do not know whether alcoholism is caused by some neurogenetic factor or by weakness of the will. Undoubtedly, both are factors. Likewise, we have only partially differentiated the spiritual from the psychological, the aesthetic from the moral, or the familial from the legal.

It is clear, however, that there is a great difference between being medically well-off and being well-off in all the other spheres in life. If the physician's task is to focus on maximizing the patient's medical well-being, he or she must realize that rational patients usually do not want their medical well-being literally maximized (at least if that comes at the price of sacrificing goods in other spheres of life). We constantly trade goods in one sphere for goods in another. We attend art shows rather than exercise classes, eat steak rather than granola—at least on occasion. If the physician's task is to try to maximize medical well-being of the patient, then wise patients will recognize that they want merely very good health, not maximum medical well-being.

This poses an enormous problem for the physician and other medical professionals. One possibility is for the physician to strive to maximize patient medical well-being. In this case, rational patients will sometimes decline to accept their doctor's advice. Maximizing medical well-being is not the same as maximizing total well-being. Moreover, if forced to choose (as we often are), surely we would rather have maximum total well-being than maximum well-being in merely one sphere of life. The rational goal (bracketing for a moment our obligations to other people) is to get our total well-being as great as possible, even if it means spending on nonmedical goods some of our time and resources that could otherwise go to making us slightly more healthy.

There is absolutely no reason to assume that the physician is skilled in making the value trade-offs between the medical and other spheres. In fact, we can predict that physicians (like experts in any other subsphere of well-being) will be biased in their recommendations. Lawyers want us to be unrealistically cautious in protecting our legal well-being. Accountants want us to keep unrealistically good financial records. Dentists want us to brush unrealistically often. And priests want us to attend religious services at unrealistic rates. So we can expect that physicians will want us to expend more of our limited resources of time, energy, and money on the medical sphere than makes sense taking into account the impacts on other spheres of life (and, therefore, on total well-being). Physicians should not be able (other than accidentally) to figure out what is truly beneficial if they concentrate exclusively on the medical.

The second possibility is for the physician to shift to a World Health Organization view that treats health as total well-being. In this case, physicians become imperialistic. They take responsibility for all aspects of life, which carries doctors well beyond their expertise. They are not equipped to promote our spiritual, legal, aesthetic, financial, or mental well-being. Physicians do not take courses in promoting our well-being by unclogging toilets, yet that is what is sometimes needed to give us total physical, mental, and social well-being.

Whether physicians view their responsibility as limited to the narrowly medical or expand their sphere to total well-being, they can be expected to fail at guessing what the proper mix ought to be between the medical and other spheres for a particular patient. In the next century this division of labor among the spheres of the good will become more important and also more complicated. As expertise in various areas becomes more complex, experts will become more specialized and their knowledge of the other spheres will correspondingly diminish. Moreover, as cultures get more and more pluralistic, we can expect people to support widely varying trade-offs among the different spheres of the good and individual physicians to be less likely to understand the value mix of any of their patients.

Why Physicians Cannot Be Expected to Know What Is Medically Beneficial

Even within the medical sphere, the problem is severe. By the mid-twentieth century the typical physician had a rather simplistic view about the nature of the medical good for his or her patients. The medical good was increasingly equated with preserving life. We had discovered antibiotics, we were aggressively pursuing polio, and we were still focused on acute illness that threatened life. The goal was to preserve life for as long as possible.

With the invention of the respirator soon after the middle of the century, physicians naturally were inclined to use it to preserve life whenever they could. Patients, however, had a much more complex view about the medical good (as did physicians of earlier centuries). They sometimes were committed to preserving life, but also desired cure of disease, relief of suffering, and, increasingly, promotion of continued good health.

This all came to a head in the case of Karen Quinlan. It became obvious that adding 10 years to her life with a respirator might not really improve even her medical well-being. Once the single-minded goal of preserving life was challenged, laypeople realized that even within the medical sphere there were many disparate goals that one could choose to pursue. Often conflicts existed among them, and no definitive method was available for balancing among these competing claims when they came into conflict. Relief of suffering might come at the expense of preserving life, preserving health at the expense of increasing pain and suffering. Keeping Karen Quinlan alive on a ventilator for 10 years was not much of a victory from the perspective of those who see little value in unconscious life.

Once again, no reason exists to assume that one's physician has a special expertise in balancing among these competing claims—even within the medical sphere. Being an expert in medicine does not make one an expert in the way the patient should make trade-offs between medical goods. In fact, as we have seen before, we have reasons to fear that physicians tend to make these medical value trade-offs atypically.

Physicians were at one point uniquely committed to preserving life. There is evidence that many of them went into medicine to fight death[3] and that they were further socialized into the death-fighting perspective once they were in the profession. These special priorities among the purposes of medicine cause physicians to make the trade-off in ways that patients would not choose. Physicians can not be expected to be able to know how to balance the competing goods even within the medical sphere. There is no such thing as a generic medical good for patients who have different priorities among the medical goods.

Why Physicians Cannot Be Expected to Know How to Balance Benefits and Harms

The problems became greater as physicians moved into the twenty-first century. Assuming, for purposes of discussion, that the physician could determine what action would maximize the medical benefit for the patient, enormous theoretical problems remain. Even before we ask whether it would be moral or legal to provide this benefit for the patient, we need to understand that the physician faces a serious problem in reconciling the Hippocratic mandate to benefit the patient with the equally Hippocratic mandate to protect the patient from harm.

Almost any medical procedure will involve a mixture of potential benefits and potential harms. Almost any procedure or drug has potential side effects. Even determining that an effect is a "side" effect rather than a "benefit" involves complex value judgments. Prevention of pregnancy by the use of a combination of estrogen and progesterone may be a tragic side effect for the Catholic woman who needs these drugs to regulate her menstrual cycle, but a cherished benefit for the woman who is trying to contracept. A priest in a Catholic country in Latin America is reported once to have claimed that these estrogen/progesterone combinations are wonderful drugs for regulating the menstrual cycle but unfortunately have the horrible side effect of preventing pregnancy. Preserving life with penicillin is wonderful for someone who wants to live, but a tragic consequence for someone with advanced metastatic cancer who wants desperately to die.

Even bracketing the fact that physicians have no expertise in determining whether an effect is beneficial or harmful (much less the degree to which it is beneficial or harmful), physicians face the even more complex task of figuring out how to balance the benefits and the harms expected from each potential treatment course. Philosophers give us many theories about how to integrate expectations of benefit and expectations of harm into a single decision.

One of the most famous approaches was advocated by British philosopher Jeremy Bentham (1748–1832), father of modern utilitarianism. Classical Benthamite utilitarians would attempt to quantify the benefits and then separately quantify the harms, after which they would subtract the harms from the benefit to arrive at an estimate of net good. Because they use addition and subtraction, this can be called an "arithmetic" approach. This, however, is not the only approach or even necessarily the most plausible.

Other utilitarians would examine the ratio of benefits to harms and opt for maximizing the size of the resulting number. This approach, called *geometric combining*, can sometimes lead to very different implications than combining benefits and harms arithmetically. If a new wonder drug has twice the potential benefit of some older remedy but also twice the risk of harm, the ratio of benefit to harm is the same, but the net benefit (that is, benefit minus harm) will be twice as large. How we judge the new drug against the old depends on which method we use to compare.

Different physicians might be inclined toward one approach or the other, yet neither is obviously correct. The physician who takes on the task of deciding what will best serve the interests of the patient must consider himself or herself authoritative in deciding which method of comparing benefits and harms is appropriate.

Consider the following example. When physicians must treat a patient with cancer, they often face a choice between a standard treatment and a more experimental one. The standard treatment typically might be seen as offering more benefit than harm, but not much of either. Although the treatment is seen as relatively safe, it is also not very effective. On the other hand, the experimental treatment might be seen as offering much more promise of cure but pose a greater threat of terrible side effects. In the interesting cases the ratio of benefits to harms is perceived to be about the same in the two treatments. If they are, that would mean that the arithmetic difference is much larger in the case of the experimental treatment. This is because both the benefits and the harms would be present in larger quantities, so subtracting the harms from the benefits must result in a larger number for the experimental treatment. Using the subtraction method, the experimental treatment is better than the standard one; using ratios (geometric comparing), the two are equally good.

The options are even more complex. Historically, some physicians entered the twentieth century committed to a corrupt variation of the Hippocratic slogan. They changed the slogan "Benefit *and* protect the patient from harm" to "First do no harm." It was sometimes rendered in Latin as *primum non nocere*. Although many physicians assume this slogan traces back to Hippocrates, neither Hippocrates nor any other Hippocratic author ever said it. (That it is in Latin rather than Greek is a warning signal.) Several of us have tried to trace this slogan's origin.[4] None of us can trace it back to either Greek or Latin medicine. I believe it dates from the mid-nineteenth century, when physicians were particularly worried about the great harm their colleagues had caused by the use of bloodletting, mercury, and other dangerous treatments. Perhaps someone rendered this concern into Latin to make it sound more profound. They said, "If we cannot help, at least we should not do harm." They elevated the avoidance of harm to the highest priority.

One interpretation is that doing no harm should come first in the sense that the physician should make sure he or she will do no harm before moving on to try to benefit the patient. This, of course, if taken literally, would have terribly conservative implications. The best way to conform would be to never do anything at all for patients. One would thereby never harm the patient (although great opportunities to do good would be lost).

For our purposes, we need to recognize that some philosophers, such as the British scholar W. D. Ross, as well as some physicians, have given the duty to avoid harming (nonmaleficence) precedence over the duty to benefit (beneficence). This might come as a special consideration given to avoiding harm, such as giving it double or triple weight when comparing harms and benefits.

It might even come as an absolute priority over beneficence—although this latter view is terribly implausible.

The point is that a physician trying to follow the Hippocratic mandate has to know how to compare benefits and harms, and there is no obvious way to go about that. Even if the physician can figure out how to relate medical benefits to overall benefits and how to relate various medical benefits to each other, there still is no reason to expect he or she will be able to know how to compare benefits and harms. The physician cannot be expected to know how to benefit the patient and protect the patient from harm. Medical ethics of the twenty-first century will have to acknowledge that this is a task beyond the ability of even the wisest, most dedicated physicians. Perhaps we will opt for the view that equates the good with patient preference or desire.[5] These theories suggest that there is no objective good in life—merely preferences or desires. In that case, however, it is hard to see why the physician's preferences or desires, rather than the patient's, should prevail. Unless physicians ask their patients, they will have no way to know.

The alternative is to accept some version of the view that the good is objective.[6] This view holds that there are some objective goods independent of preferences or desires. Even if there are objective goods and bads, however, there is absolutely no reason to believe that individual physicians have the skill for knowing what those are. There is not even any reason for believing that the consensus of physicians would be accurate in predicting what would be best for a particular patient.[7] Certainly they have the skill to predict what the effect of various treatment options will be, but they cannot know any more than an ordinary layperson whether the outcome is good or bad. If becoming a physician tends to make one atypically committed to certain kinds of goods (like staving off death), we can expect that doctors will guess wrong at what will serve the patient's interests—at least when there are several different options, each of which offers a complex mix of possible benefits and harms.

The conclusion is inescapable. Physicians cannot be expected to be able to predict what will benefit patients and protect them from harm. At best they can guess. They cannot be expected to guess correctly beyond what any ordinary citizen can. The only way physicians in the future will be able to approximate knowledge of what serves their patients' interests is to ask them.

It is not that patients will always be correct in their assessment of what is in their interests. But if they are educated with the assistance of physicians and others and become comfortable telling physicians what their interests are, the patients themselves eventually will be the most reliable sources physicians have of knowing their patients' interests.

FOUR

Sacrificing Patient Benefit to Protect Patient Rights

The insurmountable difficulties that physicians face in predicting what will benefit their patients are only the first challenge to the Hippocratic ethic that will lead to its abandonment as the new medicine becomes more and more dominant. Two other problems are even more serious. The first is deciding whether a physician who somehow knows what will maximize benefit to his or her patient should be permitted—legally or ethically—to pursue that benefit even when it violates a patient's rights. That will be our topic in this chapter. The other problem is whether a physician should pursue a patient's benefit when doing so conflicts with benefit to others. That will be the topic of the following chapter.

Around 1970 interesting cases began appearing in which it seemed that physicians should have refrained from benefiting their patients—even if they could correctly guess what would benefit them.

The Hippocratic patient-benefiting commitment strives to produce benefits and avoid harms. It deals with consequences—either good or bad. Yet in the past 30 years medical ethics has seen the reintegration of ethical perspectives into medical ethics that go beyond mere consequences. These perspectives consider ethical rights and duties as well as consequences. Although the Hippocratic ethic has always focused exclusively on consequences, many other general ethical theories have treated certain characteristics of actions other than the consequences to be morally relevant.

For example, virtually all religious traditions accept dimensions in their ethics that do not focus on consequences. Talmudic ethics is based on certain religious laws, including a prohibition on autopsy and a duty to prolong life, that are not directly based on good consequences.[1] Likewise, although Catholic natural law theory incorporates beliefs about the *telos*, or natural ends, of human beings, it is not narrowly consequentialistic.[2] Protestant ethics is usually grounded in a contract or covenant appealing to fidelity to promises rather than mere consequences.[3] Eastern religious traditions also incorporate duties not directly related to consequences, such as prohibitions on killing (of nonhuman animals as well as humans) and injunctions to truthfulness.

All fashionable secular ethical systems of the twentieth century also go beyond benefits and harms to individual patients. Classical utilitarianism requires consideration of consequences to third parties, and most other ethics incorporate notions of rights and duties not based on consequences at all. The ethical views of the German philosopher Immanuel Kant, for example, are deontological—based on duty, not consequences. According to Kant, one can have a moral duty to act in a certain way even if it does not produce the best consequences.

Liberal political philosophy produces an ethics of rights that generates certain duties to respect autonomy and promote justice. In the familiar words, it commits to liberty and justice for all. Marxism and libertarianism both abandon traditional consequentialist approaches, as does feminist ethics. The one common feature is that no plausible ethical system limits what is morally right to consequences to a single party, such as a patient. Most incorporate notions of rights and/or duties that take the ethic decidedly beyond consequences. The physician's Hippocratic ethic is utterly deviant in this regard.

The result is that these ethics, whatever their differences, all can agree that the Hippocratic commitment to benefits and harms to the patient is indefensible. Around 1970 the Hippocratic ethic of benefiting the patient was beginning to come unstuck. We discovered certain problems with benefiting the patient that have, by now, led almost everyone to abandon the Hippocratic perspective. Let's consider certain duty-based limits to benefiting patients.

The Duty to Tell the Truth

Consider first a moral issue that was very controversial in the 1960s, but is now largely settled. Imagine a patient seeing a physician for a diagnosis of a mysterious disease, which the clinician has found to be cancer. For many centuries of paternalistic medicine, the professional Hippocratic physician ethics commanded the physician to assess whether disclosure would benefit or hurt the patient. If the disclosure was thought to be helpful, the patient was to be told, but if it were deemed hurtful, it was the clinician's benevolent duty to withhold—to use a euphemism, to use jargon, or to just plain lie. In such circumstances, the consequence-driven ethic of Hippocratism instructs the physician to produce benefit or avoid harm—to use his or her judgment to protect the patient from the bad news, even though it may mean that the patient cannot plan for his or her own future, consent to medical treatment, or live the remaining days of his or her life according to an autonomously chosen life plan.

A century ago the AMA (American Medical Association) Principles of Medical Ethics was fully committed to this blatantly paternalistic approach, even at the price of serious breaches of confidentiality. That code said, "Ordinarily, the physician should not be forward to make gloomy prognostications, but should not fail, on proper occasions, to give timely notice of dangerous manifestations to the friends of the patient; even to the patient, if absolutely necessary. This notice, however, is at times so peculiarly alarming when given by the physician, that its deliverance may often be preferably assigned to another person of good judgment."[4]

The 1903 text goes on to entreat that a "solemn duty is to avoid all utterances and actions having a tendency to discourage and depress the patient."[5] The guiding Hippocratic notion was what the law called "therapeutic privilege," the doctrine that a physician has the privilege—indeed, the duty—of avoiding disclosure when telling the truth would discourage or depress the patient.

By 1980 the AMA had confronted the Kantian imperative regarding truthfulness. The tolerance of dishonesty was replaced in the rewritten 1980 code with a very simple, old-fashioned idea: The physician, without qualification, was to "deal honestly with patients and colleagues."[6] Nevertheless, the AMA's conversion to this policy of honesty was not complete. This is revealed by the AMA's Council on Ethical and Judicial Affairs when it puts its own paternalistic spin on this exceptionless pledge of honesty by saying in a 1981 interpretation that that disclosure need not be made when "risk-disclosure poses such a serious psychological threat of detriment to the patient as to be medically contraindicated."[7]

That exception, of course, is a direct contradiction of the commitment to truthfulness in the AMA's principles themselves, as well as the moral and legal requirements of duty-based systems or systems grounded in the rights of patients that are independent of consequences.

The AMA's retreat is couched in a confusing notion of "medical contraindication." This is largely meaningless. "Medicine" cannot "contraindicate" speaking the truth. All that it means is that the AMA writers believe that speaking truthfully is sometimes upsetting and that they believe the doctor is exempt from the duty to speak the truth when he or she believes the patient will be disturbed. That conclusion requires evidence that patients really are upset more by receiving the truth than by not being able to discuss a clear medical problem they may have. There is precious little evidence beyond anecdote to support the physicians' belief that they can predict harmful consequences to concealing a truthful diagnosis from a patient. Even if they can accurately predict bad consequences, patients still have a right to the facts so that they can make appropriate preparations for their future or simply so that they feel respected as mature human beings.

We now realize that in such cases, it is not so obvious that physicians should try to benefit the patient and protect the patient from harm. Some would say that the disclosure should be truthful because we now know that physicians are not very good at figuring out when a diagnosis will hurt a patient and when it will help. But more fundamentally, many take the Kantian stance that it is not right to lie and that a lie doesn't become acceptable merely because one has a benevolent motive.[8] They believe the patient has a right to the diagnosis, to form a realistic basis for consenting to future treatment, and to plan his or her future life.

One of the great contributions to ethics in the twentieth century is a book by the British philosopher W. D. Ross entitled *The Right and the Good*.[9] It proposes that there is a crucial difference between behaviors that produce good consequences and those that are morally right. Many people hold that there are certain behaviors that simply are morally right or wrong. They are right or wrong not because of their consequences, but because of their inherent characteristics. There is a formal structure to human conduct that can tend to make actions right or wrong regardless of the outcome or the consequences for the patient. One of the characteristics of actions that some people believe makes them wrong regardless of their consequences is that they contain intentional misinformation. This, of course, does not imply that all dishonest communication is always morally wrong on balance, but it does mean that some behaviors may be immoral even if, hypothetically, they would produce good consequences.

The Duty to Keep Promises

A similar claim can be made about keeping promises. One of the medical implications is in the area of confidentiality.

CONFIDENTIALITY

Imagine a physician who comes to believe that the best way he can help his patient is to disclose confidential information. One of the most important cases in the history of medical ethics involved a physician who believed that he could benefit his 16-year-old patient by disclosing to her parents that she was using birth control pills.[10] He defended his disclosure by citing the Hippocratic Oath, the British Medical Association Code of Ethics, and the Principles of the AMA, all of which suggested that it was appropriate to breach confidentiality when the physician believed it would benefit the patient. He was acquitted of the charges.

As a result of that 1970 case, medical ethics changed. From that time on, people realized it still might be wrong to break confidence even if the physician believed that doing so would benefit the patient. At least according to the new ethic for the new medicine, the physician has the duty to inform the patient that the confidence is being broken. Most of us believe that if the patient does not give permission, the information cannot be disclosed. That is not what the Hippocratic Oath says. The Oath states merely that the physician should not disclose "that which should not be spoken abroad," implying that some things should be spoken abroad—such as information that the physician feels could benefit the patient. That old Hippocratic interpretation was incorporated into the old AMA and British codes for physicians, but most of us now reject it. Even the medical professional associations have changed their codes so as to require keeping such information confidential unless the patient gives permission for disclosure.

KEEPING OTHER PROMISES

Similarly, many believe that there is a moral duty to keep promises other than the promise of confidentiality—and to keep them regardless of the consequences. When physicians promise to stay with patients during a critical medical crisis, they have a duty to do so even if they come to believe that they could do more good if they transferred responsibility to other caregivers. Of course, if the patient consents to the changing or abandoning of the promise, the physician is released, but the mere fact that the doctor could do more good for the patient by breaking a promise does not automatically justify breaking it. Once again, there are times when it is morally wrong for the physician to do what will benefit the patient.

The Duty to Respect Autonomy

The 1970s gave us a third example of cases in which physicians are expected to refrain from doing what they think would benefit their patient, the most prominent of which involved patients or their families who tried to refuse life-supporting medical treatment. Literally hundreds of patients were trapped by their doctors, condemned to receive medical treatments just because their physicians believed it was beneficial.

Even in cases in which there are no violations of perceived moral duties, some patients may decline certain benefits that have been offered them. In some of these cases, a disagreement exists between the physician and patient about whether the proposed treatment will really benefit the patient. In other cases, the patient may agree that the treatment should count as a benefit and still want to decline it. Consider a terminally ill cancer patient who is told that a long and expensive course of chemotherapy, which would involve considerable burdens on family members, has a modest chance of benefit. Some people may conclude that it is in their interests to receive the therapy but nevertheless not want to accept the offer because it conflicts with the interests of certain family members (by consuming resources or imposing caregiving burdens).

If a patient decides to reject a proposed benefit in order to advance the interests of loved ones, it seems clear that the oncologist should refrain from benefiting this patient. Some might argue that such treatments really won't benefit patients because patients would feel guilty over burdens imposed on their families. In that case, the treatment does not really benefit the patients on balance. In other cases, though, patients may want to refuse not because they will feel guilty, but rather because they just think it is the right thing to do. Treating in the face of a refusal of treatment is not only a violation of patient autonomy, it is also a violation of the reasonable ethic of permitting people to make self-sacrifice in order to express their loyalty to their familial community.

Respect for individuals' autonomy is the most well-rehearsed discussion of the way in which late-twentieth century medical ethics departs from the earlier paternalistic Hippocratism. We have even become accustomed to permitting people to make foolish choices that conflict with their own interests as well as the interests of others. As long as the patient is mentally competent and understands the choices he or she is making, it is the doctor's duty to respect the patient's refusal of treatment. Only when the patient has been found mentally incompetent would we intervene. In those cases, there is no patient autonomy to respect.

But what of cases in which the patient, perhaps through confusion or error, chooses to decline a beneficial treatment for reasons other than these? Many defenders of patient autonomy believe that the patient may know his own interests better than the physician. But that is not always the case. There surely are at least a few situations in which the doctor really does know best. If those situations, no matter how rare, can be identified, then the ethic of doing what is best for the patient would not only permit, but actually require, that the physician act on his or her judgment.

Even in these cases, however, many believe that the patient has the right to act autonomously to refuse the offer of treatment. The patient has a right to act foolishly. If that is true, it would be morally wrong for the physician to benefit the patient in these cases as well. Usually doctors do not know best—and even when they do, they should refrain from benefiting the competent patient who doesn't want the benefit. The duty to respect autonomy has its real bite when there is good reason to believe that the physician really can help the patient by violating his or her autonomy. Those committed to autonomy, including anyone standing in the tradition of liberal political philosophy, will insist that the physician has a duty not to benefit the patient in these cases.

The Duty to Avoid Killing

It is possible that some very sick people actually could be better off dead. If the Hippocratic Oath requires the physician to act so as to benefit the patient, why should the physician not act to put a patient out of her misery? If there is no other way to relieve severe, intractable suffering, why not kill the patient?

One interpretation of Hippocratic ethics is that patient-benefit ethics does indeed lead to that conclusion. The duty of the physician, they claim, is to relieve the suffering by killing the patient or helping the patient kill herself. That is Jack Kevorkian's view.[11] Others follow another provision in the Oath that prohibits physician participation in active killing even if it would produce a net improvement in the patient's well-being. Whether it is implied in the Hippocratic Oath, it is widely held that there is simply something wrong with the intentional killing of humans. Catholics, Jews, Hindus, Buddhists, and Muslims, as well as proponents of mainstream secular liberal political philosophy, have traditionally believed that active mercy killing is morally wrong, even if the consequences are good. Not everyone accepts this constraint on producing good for patients, but many people do.

Rights and Duties Forbid Benefit to the Patient

The foregoing were four examples of situations that by the 1970s caused us to struggle with the old Hippocratic idea that the physician's sole moral duty is to benefit the patient. Patients have rights and because of that, physicians have duties that sometimes forbid doing not only what they think will benefit their patients, but also what actually will be beneficial. During that first phase of what I call the "new medicine," many came to believe it would be wrong for a physician to do what would benefit the patient, even if the physician could successfully identify what that would be. Physicians were, according to these limits, required to speak honestly, keep promises, respect autonomy, and avoid killing. Thus, the second reason why physicians of the new medicine must stop trying to benefit patients is that virtually every moral system that is at all plausible incorporates at least some of these limits on patient benefit.

So far we have discovered that it is normally very hard, indeed often impossible, for the physician to know what to do to benefit patients and protect them from harm. We have also found that even if they could figure this out, the rights of patients will sometimes forbid offering this benefit. There is one final, particularly serious, problem with setting out to benefit patients: Sometimes the interests of others will conflict. The next chapter sets out this final, critical problem with the ethic of benefiting patients.

FIVE | Societal Interests and Duties to Others

This brings us to the third and final reason why physicians in the twenty-first century will have to stop trying to benefit patients. Almost every plausible ethical system other than the Hippocratic one acknowledges that legitimate societal interests impinge on the patient-physician relation. We are not as far along in recognizing this third problem, but most scholars in medical ethics by now understand that there are times when the patient's interest must be sacrificed for the good of society or to fulfill duties to others.

Sacrificing Patient Benefit to Serve the Interests of Others in Society

Classical social utilitarianism tries to produce the best possible consequences, *taking into account the interests of all parties potentially affected*. If the duty-based ethics of respect for autonomy was the challenge to Hippocratic ethics of the late twentieth century, then the social ethics requiring consideration of the interests and/or rights of other parties is surely the challenge of the twenty-first century. We are moving into a period when virtually everyone who is thoughtful will eventually recognize that an ethic that permits each physician to do whatever would serve the best interest of his or her patient would be a grossly irresponsible ethic. It would not only permit, but would require, lying, cheating, and stealing from the health insurance system in order to serve the patient. It would require that physicians use scarce medical resources for the benefit of their own patients, even if the benefit to them was infinitesimally small and the cost to others tremendous. The Hippocratic ethic, taken literally, would require the physician to do whatever he or she could to bring any possible benefit to the patient, no matter how small the benefit. That seems to require that physicians spend nights sitting by their patients' bedsides if only that might help the patient. Physicians would have to ignore other obligations: to their family, their colleagues, future patients, and themselves. No reasonable person would expect physicians to do this, especially if other patients would be harmed in the process.

The Hippocratic ethic is an utterly individualistic ethic. It is as if there were only one patient in the world and one physician, and the physician's task was to maximize the interests of the patient. But in the real world, there are other patients. There are also nonpatients who have interests, some of which may be legitimate. The final challenge to the medical ethics of the twenty-first century is to develop a social ethic for medicine that addresses the hyperindividualism of the Hippocratic tradition without capriciously sacrificing the individual patient to the vicissitudes of social utility.

Sacrificing the Patient to Fulfilling Duties to Others

Working out that responsible social ethic for medicine will be one of the great projects of the next century. It cannot possibly be resolved here. Nevertheless, I think we already have a hint of what it will look like.

At the level of individual ethics, we overcame the consequentialism of the Hippocratic tradition by appealing to certain duties or rights that provided limited justifications for abandoning patient benefit. I suggest that the same strategy will lead to the resolution of the conflict between the interests of the individual and the interests of society. We will find that the conflict is resolved by recognizing that certain claims of others in society against the rights and interests of the individual patients are legitimate, whereas others are not. The legitimating feature will be found in other ethical principles rather than maximizing good consequences, principles such as promise keeping, honesty, and, most important, justice.

DUTIES OF PROMISE KEEPING

I list promise keeping first because the structure of the moral analysis is relatively simple, although it is unlikely to occur often in practice. The idea is quite simple: One justifying reason for abandoning the patient is that a legitimate promise has been made to someone else that interferes with treating the patient.

CASE 5.1

A Kidney for Your Patient

A physician has a patient who needs a kidney transplant. He also knows that a brain-dead patient is currently in the hospital. The physician realizes he might try to benefit his patient by persuading the family of that brain-dead patient to donate a kidney directly to his patient needing the kidney. Such directed donations are legal according to the National Organ Transplant Act. But the physician has committed himself to a policy of organ allocation based on the national computerized formula that attempts to distribute kidneys as efficiently and equitably as possible. He knows that even though his particular patient won't get the kidney, in the long run the overall system will be better for patients in general. Moreover, he knows that it will be a more fair arrangement.

If he has committed himself to the national allocation system, then he would be breaking his promise if he tried to circumvent the national system to get an organ donated directly to his patient. Getting the donation directed to his patient would probably be best for his patient. If he pursued only patient benefit, he would try to get the family to donate directly to that patient. However, if he had made the promise to play by the national allocation rules and didn't want to break his promise, he would have to refrain from pursuing the directed donation.

DUTIES OF HONESTY

Second, consider the classic cases of gaming the insurance system in order to benefit the patient. A physician realizes that her patient needs a medical procedure that she cannot afford. The insurance company will not cover the procedure if it is described honestly, but would cover it if a deceptive, equivocal diagnosis were given.

A Pap Smear for Nervous Nellie

For example, the insurer might not cover a routine Pap smear for Nellie Nickerson, a nervous, cancer-phobic 45-year-old worried that she may have cancer, but would cover it if her physician describes it to the insurer as a test to "rule out cancer." The Pap smear would make the patient feel better and carries essentially no risk. It seems it is in the patient's interest for the physician to mislead the insurance company in order to get the test paid for. It is, of course, contrary to the interests of the insurance company. More importantly, it is also contrary to the interests of the other subscribers. The Hippocratic ethic requires lying or deceiving here (because it requires doing what would benefit the patient). A study of physicians has shown that most physicians in this kind of case would try to deceive the insurer.[1] However, the physician might decide it is morally appropriate to refrain from deceiving. She might even do so without adopting a purely social utilitarian ethic. She might merely acknowledge the moral principle of veracity—that it is morally required that she act truthfully.

In this case, as in the transplant example, the physician may decide to sacrifice her patient and act in a socially responsible way *without adopting social utility as the basis*. Fidelity to promises and veracity open the door to very limited patient sacrifice without opening the floodgates of social utilitarianism.

DUTIES OF JUSTICE

By far the most important way of moving in the direction of a social ethic is to incorporate a principle of justice into a medical ethic. A principle of justice would provide a way of considering some social claims while ruling out others. It could do so without basing the decision on the principle of maximizing social consequences. That will sometimes permit the physician to sacrifice the patient at the margin and lead to serving societal interests without adopting the principle of social utility.

Justice is a principle that recognizes the legitimacy of certain patterns of distribution of good other than those that will maximize the net good in aggregate. Depending on the type of pattern one supports, it could lead to distribution based on (as Aristotle puts it) noble birth, free birth, or excellence.[2] In the twenty-first century the dominant basis for a just distribution is *need*. According to this egalitarian notion of justice, distributions are morally just insofar as they arrange resources on the basis of how poorly off people are or on the basis of what actions are necessary to make people more equal.[3]

Why We Shouldn't Distribute Kidneys Efficiently

The national organ transplant system in the United States is formally committed to promoting justice (or what it calls equity) as well as producing the greatest amount of good with the limited supply of organs for transplant. It turns out that the best way to get as much good as possible from the organs would be to distribute them in a manner that would be blatantly unfair. Men, for example, do slightly better with some transplants. (At least historically they did before we got better at blocking rejection.) For kidneys, because of some complex factors related to tissue compatibility, Caucasians have done slightly better than Blacks and other minorities.[4] The best way to get as much good as possible from the transplant system would be to give all the organs to Caucasian males. We are not about to do that—and we shouldn't. It would be grossly unfair. Especially because the differences are very small, we want a public system of organ allocation to also consider fairness. Physicians are morally obliged not only to avoid doing everything that would help their patients on the waiting list for organs, they are also obliged to refrain from giving all the organs to the people who would get the most benefit (measured in terms of survival of the organ graft or the patient.

We want a health-care system that is fair, and that means intentionally avoiding doing everything that could benefit either the patient or the social group as a whole. This suggests a basis for a limited strategy for sacrificing individual patients at the margin. The patient might be seen as having no entitlement to a scarce medical resource when there are others with greater need could use that resource).

Of course, a full theory of health-care justice would be exceedingly complex. I have advocated allocating certain high-tech, experimental, life-prolonging technologies on this basis, but a more complete theory must be left to the ethicists of the next century to create. The point is that if the hyperindividualistic Hippocratic ethic is to be replaced with a more social ethic that requires certain compromises with patient interests, then some basis for limiting that social ethic will be needed. I suggest that the key is in limiting the sacrifice of the patient to those cases in which some duty other than maximizing good consequences in the aggregate provides a justification—whether that principle be fidelity to promises, veracity, or justice. An alternative—which I consider, but reject—would be to balance these duty-based obligations against the amount of aggregate good. That is the method suggested by W. D. Ross,[5] as well as many contemporary medical ethicists,[6] but I find that this approach poses serious risks to well-established rights and leads to conclusions that are contrary to considered moral judgments. Regardless of where someone comes out on that debate, everyone must agree that it would be wrong to turn physicians loose to do whatever would most benefit their own patients.

SIX

The New, Limited, Twenty-First-Century Role for Physicians as Patient Assistants

Limiting Physicians from Benefiting Patients

The previous three chapters have provided a three-pronged analysis for why physicians must stop trying to benefit their patients. First, they cannot know what will benefit patients because reasonable patients have interests beyond the health. All rational people will make marginal sacrifices of their medical well-being in order to pursue other dimensions of a good life. Even within the medical sphere, there is no such thing as a single medical good. Saving lives, curing disease, relieving suffering, and promoting continued health are all worth pursuing, but striving for one will sometimes come at the expense of one of the other components of medical well-being. There is no definitively correct way to trade off one aspect of medical well-being for another. The right balance will depend on individual, subjective preferences, and physicians cannot know what the right balance is for their patients without asking them.

Second, benefiting the patient will sometimes come at the price of sacrificing what we owe to others. Patients may not want their interests pursued because they are worried about those of family members or friends. Or physicians may be required by the moral principles of fidelity to promises, autonomy, veracity, and avoidance of killing to back off and intentionally refrain from striving to benefit the patient.

Finally, trivial benefits for the patient may be purchased at the price of losing much greater good for society and, more important, may come only by violating our duty to treat people fairly.

Exempting Physicians from Social Ethics

Having said this, it may turn out to be a mistake to instruct physicians to abandon their patients whenever others have stronger claims of justice to resources. It is deeply troublesome to contemplate a patient-physician relation in which the physician is expected to sacrifice the patient whenever social utility or justice calls for it. It would require the physician to take down the Hippocratic Oath plaque from the waiting room wall and replace it with a sign reading, "Warning, all ye who enter here. I have been asked by society to abandon you at the margin and serve society as its cost-containment agent."

There may be something left of the sacredness of the patient-physician relation that requires continued loyalty of the clinician to the patient, even in the face of legitimate societal claims of justice for the resources to be used elsewhere.

I think an alternative may emerge in the new medicine: Physicians could be given a limited exemption from the societal obligation to promote justice in the allocation of resources. They would be charged with the duty of loyalty to their patients while in the patient-physician relation. They would, in effect, be expected to be more like defense attorneys. They would be loyal to their patients while expecting other people in other roles to watch out for the interests and rights of other parties. Just as the defense attorney expects the plaintiff's attorney and the judge and jury to combine to achieve a fair outcome, so the clinician might be expected to remain loyal to her patient while expecting other health professionals, administrators, and public officials to make sure that the patient does not consume too much of the community's medical resources.

CASE 6.1

Livers and Money in HMOs

A 39-year-old man came to an appointment with his HMO internist after routine tests revealed he had abnormal liver function. Further tests revealed he had a mass in his liver that was cancerous. By the time it was diagnosed it had grown to 5 cm in diameter.

This was bleak news. The only treatment was a liver transplant, but if the tumor had metastasized so that cells were growing outside the liver, the transplant would do no good. Because the early metastases were not detectable clinically, judgment had to be made about whether a transplant was justified on the basis of the size of the mass in the liver. Most transplant centers consider 5 cm diameter to be the upper limit of whether a transplant is justified.

The patient's internist consulted with the transplant center with which the HMO had a contract for all transplant surgery. That program would refuse to operate on the patient. This left the internist with a dilemma about what to say to her patient. She finally said simply, "You are not a candidate for transplant."

In fact, there were two other centers in the United States that were, on an experimental basis, transplanting livers for persons with primary liver cancer. The prognosis for such surgery was not good. The patient would have less than 10 percent chance of surviving. The cost of the surgery would be $200,000. Because it was estimated that only 1 in 10 would survive, that calculated to $2,000,000 per life saved. We know that in one sense, human life is priceless, but that is much more than our society normally spends to save lives in other areas such as highway safety. Put another way, if someone had $2,000,000 available, they could save several lives if they spent the money some way other than on a transplant for someone with a 5-cm growth in his liver.

Before the internist told the patient he was not a candidate, she had consulted with the medical director of the HMO, the one who makes final decisions about authorizing controversial and expensive procedures. The medical director understood that the patient could go to one of the experimental programs and that the HMO could pay the bill. He claimed that he thought it would be a waste of organs to use one of these scarce, precious, life-saving organs on someone who had only a 10 percent chance. On that basis, he refused to approve the transplant and the internist gave the patient the deceptively vague news that he was not a candidate.

This poor patient died about a year later. He died in spite of the fact that had he known, there was a chance—a small chance—that he could have been saved. It turns out that this patient was quite wealthy. He invested in oil and could have considered paying for the operation out of his own pocket had he understood what it meant when he was told he was not a candidate for the transplant.

His internist and the medical director of the HMO both played controversial roles in this case. A good argument can be made that they both abused the duties of their roles. The problem with the internist's performance is perhaps more obvious. She took on a patient with an implied pledge that she would work for his benefit. She could have told him that although the HMO's contracted transplant center would not agree to a transplant, two other places in the United States would consider it. She could have told him that he had only a 10 percent chance of surviving with the surgery, but no chance without it. She could have played the role of the patient advocate in this case, petitioning her medical director for authorization to have the HMO cover the transplant outside of its normal contract.

A good case can be made that she should have lost in her fight for her patient, but she could have fought for him. Perhaps she should have lost because $2,000,000 of the HMO's resources to save one life is a very large investment. Even if this were a nonprofit, patient-owned HMO, it is not clear that the members would agree to such expenditures. There must be some limit on what is spent of a group's funds. Reasonable members of an HMO may say that $2,000,000 is too high a price. Put another way, they may have said, "If my premium is going to increase by my share of that $2,000,000 in order to save other people's lives, I would rather spend that money more efficiently saving more lives in the process. I will contribute to refugee food programs or flu vaccine programs, either of which would save many more lives."

If some amount is too high a price for a life saved in an HMO and the internist is going to be an advocate for the patient who needs the transplant in order to have a chance to live, then someone else in the HMO needs to be the one looking out for the other members. A good case can be made that that person should be the medical director or someone else in a management role whose job it is to look out for the interests of the community as a whole.

The medical director could have said that he would not approve the experimental transplant at HMO expense because it was an irresponsible use of a large amount of the community's money. He could have rejected the petition and denied the coverage. Interestingly, had he done so, the patient could have been told by the internist the real reason for the denial. He could have been told about the 10 percent chance and how much of the HMO resources that would consume. Had he been told the truth, the patient, independently wealthy, could have then decided whether he wanted to pay for the surgery himself and have a small but real chance of surviving. The internist would have fulfilled her duty to be a loyal advocate for the patient. She would have lost, but she would have remained loyal. In the process, the patient would have known the truth and would have avoided having his only chance to live denied him.

There could have been a moral division of labor between the internist, who could have been the patient advocate, and the medical director, who would have had a duty to keep an eye on the interests of the group. Instead, the internist abandoned her patient by couching the denial in ambiguous terms that made it sound like the patient had no option. In the meantime, the medical director also abandoned his role. Instead of looking out for the welfare of the HMO community, he took it upon himself to guard the organ pool. He claimed he was worried about a national concern—wasting an organ on someone with only a small chance of surviving—when he could have said he was worrying about the interests of his HMO community. In fact, the responsible allocation of organs is the job of others, the personnel of the United Network for Organ Sharing (UNOS), the national organ procurement and transplantation network assigned this task by the federal government. The members of UNOS are well aware of their responsibility to use organs judiciously. Part of carrying out that responsibility includes assigning some small number of these precious commodities to research programs such as those at the two centers that were researching a potential life-saving operation for people now destined to die.

The medical director of the HMO was in a poor position to decide whether the organ was being used wastefully. He was in a good position to decide about the use of the HMO's resources. The internist was in a poor position to monitor the allocation of HMO resources. She could not know how the $200,000 that might be spent on this patient would otherwise be used. If she was intentionally vague in telling this patient about his options in order to cover for the HMO's decision, she was abandoning her proper role just as surely as the medical director was when he refused to base his decision on the money involved. A moral division of labor may be the only way our society can use resources responsibly while still leaving clinicians free to play their more traditional role as advocates for their patients. In this case, it may have cost a patient his life.

The New Role for Physicians as Patient Assistants

If this moral division of labor is adopted, clinical caregivers would pledge to work always for the benefit of the patient within three constraints. The first constraint would be the knowledge that the only way they can reliably know the patient's interest is to ask the patient. Thus, they would not follow the Hippocratic dictum to work for the patient's interest according to the *physician's* ability and judgment, but rather according to the *patient's* ability and judgment. In this sense, physicians and other health professionals should be reconceptualized as assistants for patients who can provide critical help providing information about the facts of their diagnoses, explanation and advice about the treatment options available, and advocacy in negotiating a complex, alien system called health care.

The second constraint would be that of the duty-based principles. Clinical caregivers sometimes would be permitted to refrain from serving the patient's interests in order to avoid breaking promises (including promises of confidentiality), telling lies (including lies about diagnosis and prognosis), violating respect for patient autonomy, or killing (even killing the patient when it is in the patient's interest).

The third constraint will be the most difficult to articulate. I suggest that clinicians should promise their patients that they will always remain loyal in informing them about treatment options and providing those options chosen by the patient subject to two limits: The physician should not be forced to violate unjustly his or her own conscience and should not be permitted to use resources in ways that violate the just claims of others who are in greater need.

Hence, the physician can say to the 45-year-old patient whose interests will be served by the Pap smear, "I promise to advise you about all your options (including the test that is not covered by your insurance policy) and do everything in my power to follow the course you choose. I cannot, however, lie for you to get the test covered. Moreover, even though I will fight for you to get the test at the insurer's expense, it may be that the insurer has morally just reasons for setting limits that I can do nothing about. I will remain loyal to you as your agent and assistant in procuring what you believe are your medical interests, but, in the end, I may lose."

That is the role I also envision for the internist assisting the patient with liver cancer. She should have advocated for and assisted her patient in getting what he believes will serve his interest. She should fight for the HMO funding of the transplant, but probably she should lose. When she loses, it will be because other physicians who are not in a clinical care giving role have fulfilled their role-specific obligation to do what is moral from the institutional perspective. When the internist loses, she still is in a position to advocate for and assist the patient in exploring whether he wants to seek the experimental procedure at his own expense.

This would be a radically different role for the physician than that of one that saw the clinician balancing the patient's interests against those of the society. It would mean that the decisions about the just claims of society against the patient's well-being are adjudicated not by the physician, but by others—presumably a democratic process in which the patient participated. I will have more to say about how patients can participate actively in setting health insurance limits in chapters 16 and 17. The physician in the clinical role would be completely exempt from any obligation to suggest limits on the patient's well-being, even at the margin. Instead, the physician would always (within the constraints of the difficulties of determining patient interest and the deontological obligations previously discussed) pursue the patient's interests, but know that he or she is working in a just system in which often, at the margin, he or she will lose to other claims that are more just.

One thing is clear: Medical ethics in the next century will be radically different from the outmoded, anachronistic, paternalistic, individualistic ethic attributed to Hippocrates. It will acknowledge that physicians normally cannot be expected to figure out on their own what will benefit their patients and that often they should not try to provide such benefits, even if they can figure them out. Although many people, especially theorists in medical ethics, increasingly have a vague understanding of this insight, almost no one yet has yet realized that it means that literally every decision a physician makes—the pattern of every practice—will have to be altered radically. It will mean that in every patient-physician encounter, it will no longer make sense for physicians to prescribe, certify "medical necessity," or even recommend any treatment, let alone give "orders" or claim they know what is best for the patient. Figuring out why these old concepts will no longer work and what new terms must be used in their place in what we are calling the new medicine is the project of the next chapters.

SEVEN

Abandoning Modern Medical Concepts

Doctor's "Orders" and Hospital "Discharge"

If a new medicine is on the horizon, a new language will be needed. The old terms of modern medicine will no longer do. The civil rights and women's movements sensitized us to the offensiveness of our standard, old language. We can no longer, in good conscience, refer to a Black man as a "boy" or a woman as a "girl" (or sometimes even a "lady"). We can no longer with innocence use the masculine pronouns as surrogates for gender-neutral terms. Linguistic conventions that worked well in a former era are offensive once we realize that the old assumptions are indefensible.

Just as the civil rights and women's movements taught us that the old language contained indefensible assumptions, so in the new medicine we will discover that in health care, too, the old way of talking is anachronistic. We will no longer, with a straight face, be able to speak of "doctor's orders" and "discharge from the hospital." I tackle these terms in this chapter. In the two that follow I will take on "medically indicated treatments," "treatments of choice," or even of "medical necessity."

Doctor's "Orders": The Doctor Is Not a Military General

The active participation of patients (and patient surrogates) in medical decision making is grounded on the notion that values from outside medicine must control medical decisions. Patients are the primary persons with the skill to decide what is good medicine, because they are usually the ones who best know what will maximize their own well-being. Even in cases in which a patient does not know best, he or she still bears certain rights of decision making grounded in the principle of autonomy.

I sometimes refer to this as the "partnership model" of the patient-physician relation.[1] The patient is in an active partnership with the physician in working out what will serve the patient's interest. It is not really an equal partnership because the focus is on the medical and other interests of the patient. Thus, the patient is the senior partner or the managing partner. The physician is present in the relation to provide assistance to the patient in areas in which the patient lacks adequate skills or knowledge. Sometimes that will require the physician to make decisions—to decide what subjects to bring up with the patient and to outline all the tests or treatment options that are at all plausible (even if some of them offend the physician's sense of what is appropriate). The final choices will, for the most part, however, rest with the patient. Even in cases in which the patient is a child or a mentally compromised adult, some surrogate for the patient—a parent, spouse, or someone holding a power of attorney—will be the one deciding on the patient's behalf, not the physician. In those rare cases in which surrogates have to be overruled because they are acting irresponsibly—foolishly or maliciously—it will be some other authority, such as a judge, that overrules the surrogate. The physician's role will be secondary in the sense that he or she might have to be the person who determines if a valid surrogate is available or asks for judicial intervention to overrule the primary decision maker. Thus, the patient (or patient's agent) is the primary decision maker and the physician the secondary one.

This partnership approach to decision making poses serious problems for certain key concepts and terms used in traditional Hippocratic modern medicine. One of the most common and problematic is the notion of "doctor's orders." This term is pervasive in medical usage—accepted by layperson and clinician alike—even though it implies authority and decision-making relations that no longer make sense.

One of the most common places in which the term *orders* appears is the "do not resuscitate order." The "do not resuscitate order" has become an important phenomenon in the evolution of more responsive and humane care of critically and terminally ill patients. Guidelines for decisions pertaining to resuscitation have been developed and are the source of much research,[2] therapeutic discussion,[3] and policy debate.[4]

Why does an institution as important as health care choose the image of order giver? That language conflicts with a movement in society and the health professions alike toward a consensual, or covenantal, model in which the patient makes choices with the support of significant others including family, friends, clergy, and health-care professionals.

We are at a point at which we will have to choose among competing models for structuring the relation between the health professional and the layperson. One model, what I have called the "priestly model," is a residuum from the day when medicine was viewed as the realm of experts with the authority that comes from possessing potent, secret wisdom. It is an authoritarian model in which decisions rest on the authority of the expert. In medicine they even have a name for this special dominance. They call it "Aesculapian authority," referring to the Greek god of medicine.

This priestly model stands in contrast with the partnership, or contract, model, which emphasizes cooperation between physicians and patients toward the common goals of disease treatment, disease prevention, and health promotion.

It is hard to escape the conclusion that the language of order giving had its origins in and fits best with the priestly model. The question then is whether it is meaningful or appropriate for the newer, more cooperative approach to decision making. Part of the controversy stems from the fact that the word *order* is used in two very different ways. "Doctor's orders" in the first sense fits best with the more traditional, authoritarian model. The orders are authoritative instructions based on the physician's judgment about what is in the patient's best interest. For matters such as ordering resuscitation or ordering its omission, in which the choice is heavily contingent on the patient's own beliefs and values, the decision should not be based on the practitioner's judgment. That is why most of the formal guidelines on resuscitation have insisted that the choice belongs to the patient.

Why, then, do the guidelines on resuscitation (and many of the commentators) still speak of orders? It must be that the term is being used in a newer, more sophisticated way. Some say that *orders* is being used, without authoritarian overtones, as the standard term for all communication from physicians—including communications of the patient's judgment about whether care is accepted or refused. The physicians then are not ordering on their own; they are transmitting the patient's choice (the patient's orders).

But this sounds like a rationalization for a term that clearly came from a more command-oriented world. Is that the right term for the newer, more cooperative era in which patients are viewed as more active decision makers?

Many professions rely on authoritative transmission of instructions without giving orders. Business professionals do not speak of giving orders to their staffs; researchers do not talk of giving orders to their research teams. They ask, request, say "please," and adopt other subtleties of respectful speech, even when it is understood by all that such requests are to be carried out. Only physicians and military officers still speak of giving orders. Why is it, then, that physicians—even if they are only transmitting decisions patients have made about accepting or refusing care—are so firmly attached to the language of order giving? It is just inappropriate to use such language in the newer, more cooperative model of the patient-physician partnership.

"Discharge": The Hospital Is Not a Prison

Similar funny, but troublesome, language creeps into hospital vocabulary. A particularly vivid example occurred in the days after the president was shot.

CASE 7.1

Discharging the Supreme Commander

> On the afternoon of March 30, 1981, President Ronald Reagan was leaving the Washington Hilton when six shots rang out that left him hospitalized at the George Washington Hospital. Fortunately, he recovered and soon was handling some presidential responsibilities from the hospital. The press briefing duties at the hospital were handled by Dr. Dennis O'Leary. By Tuesday, April 7, he was saying that Reagan would be "released" from the hospital and return to the White House early in the week. By that Saturday, he was hoping that the president "probably will be discharged today." It actually was not until the next day that O'Leary was quoted as saying, "We are quite comfortable letting him go home today."

The doctor's language was remarkable. President Reagan was arguably the most powerful human being on the face of the earth, the commander-in-chief for Americans, yet doctors—ones with no historical ties to the president—could talk about releasing him, discharging him, and letting him go home. At first, it might seem that deciding when he should leave the hospital was a "medical" decision. Surely, the doctors were experts on the risks of going home too early and even the risks of staying too long. But more careful thought makes it apparent how wrong that way of thinking is. Surely, there is a time at the beginning of the hospital stay when almost no one would choose to leave. Granted, they force mothers of newborns out the door within 24 hours. The hernia patient in chapter 2 wasn't even allowed to stay overnight. The length of stay also can be too long, when the risk of picking up an iatrogenic (hospital-induced) infection would outweigh any value of staying in the hospital. But the real question, especially in the case of the president of the United States, is how important it is for him to be at the White House. On the one hand, he may have critical decisions to make that can be handled only in his office. On the other hand, he certainly has assistants to bring him work in the hospital. In the end, deciding how long the president should stay is not something that Dr. O'Leary or any of his colleagues should be able to know, at least without understanding how important it is for the president to leave and what burdens he will suffer once he returns to his home environment. At most, they might be able to advise the president on the medical risks of leaving the hospital on various days.

Even more puzzling than the assumption that doctors could know when it was proper for the president to leave the hospital was the language they used. It was vintage hospital talk: discharge, release, let go. It is language more fitting for the military or a prison. It takes a certain chutzpah to talk that way about discharging the president. Even though we know, at a certain level, that this is only doctor-talk, the presumptions it implies are deeply troublesome.

Why do hospitals and doctors adopt the language of the military and the prison? Surely, it is because they presume custody and control in a manner analogous to those authoritarian institutions. Even as metaphors they are troubling. In more recent times the patient's right to leave against the decision of the doctor is recognized, but it is often termed "signing out against medical advice." That one would have to sign out, presumably signing some sort of release from liability, is quite amazing. No other professionals, to my knowledge, would claim the authority to discharge or release a client. None would require the client to sign a release form to leave against the professional's advice.

Imagine, for example, a member of the clergy counseling a parishioner who decides she wants to end the session and leave. How would she respond if the priest insisted she could not leave without signing a release? Or consider one of my students stopping by my office to discuss a term paper, only to be told he could not leave without signing a form releasing me from liability.

Ronald Reagan apparently got some revenge. On the day he finally left, according to the *Washington Post*, "In accord with hospital rules Reagan was wheeled to the elevator, but he said, 'I walked in here. I'm going to walk out,' and left his wheelchair behind."

The policy of requiring patients to leave the hospital in wheelchairs is a very strange one. If a doctor is asked, he or she will likely claim it is to protect the hospital from liability in case the patient should fall. That doesn't make much sense, however. My advice is that when one is told that he must be pushed out in a wheelchair, the proper question is, "Doctor, in your professional opinion, am I able to walk or not?" If the doctor says you are able to walk, then you might as well do so. If he says you are not able, then you should ask how you are supposed to get around once outside the hospital door. Upon reflection, if there is fear the patient may collapse if he walks, it makes much more sense for that to occur on the hospital floor where there are skilled professionals ready to intervene. If the patient first walks on his own after returning to his home, the collapse will occur in the privacy of a residence where no one is available to help. As a matter of principle, people who are going to walk as soon as they go out the door of the hospital should walk to the door, not be pushed.

The language of doctor's orders and hospital discharges is a telltale sign of outdated thinking of the old-fashioned modern medicine. Another cluster of concepts is similarly revealing. When we speak of "medically indicated treatment," "treatment of choice," or "medically necessary treatment," we are trying to dress up our value judgments in a scientific aura that cannot survive in the revealing environment of postmodern medicine. These terms will be our focus in the next two chapters.

| Medicine Can't "Indicate"

So Why Do We Talk That Way?

The notion of doctor's orders is problematic in a partnership model of medical decision making. Doctors use another set of term that is even more problematic. They talk about certain drugs or treatments being "medically indicated," certain treatments being "treatments of choice," and under certain circumstances procedures such as abortion or withdrawal of life support being "medically necessary." This odd talk needs to be exposed so that we see it for what it is: attempts to clothe value judgments in medicine with a garb of medical objectivity.

"Medically Indicated Treatment"? Medicine Can't Tell Us Which Drugs to Use

Doctors, textbook writers, and Food and Drug Administration officials all love to use the term "medically indicated treatment." To say a drug is "indicated" for a particular condition is just an obscure way of saying it is appropriate or good for that condition. An antibiotic is said to be "indicated" for a bacterial infection if the antibiotic will treat that infection. Drug manufacturers and the FDA talk about a drug's "indications" when they simply mean its recommended uses.

Like doctor's orders, the notion of a treatment's being medically indicated is built on an understanding of medical decision making that incorporates assumptions that are no longer tenable in a postmodern world of a new medicine. The implication of claiming that a drug is medically indicated is simply that by knowing medical science well, a practitioner can determine the appropriate treatment for a patient, independent of the patient's beliefs, values, and commitments.

At the center of the partnership model of the new medicine is the realization that it is literally impossible to know what good medicine is without knowing whether an intervention furthers the rights and well-being of the patient, and it is impossible to know whether these are advanced without involving the patient actively in the decision-making process. The literature on the "do not resuscitate" order, which so comfortably makes use of the notion of doctor's orders, also incorporates the notion of medically indicated treatment.

The Report of the 1985 National Conference on Standards and Guidelines for Cardiopulmonary Resuscitation and Emerging Cardiac Care states that "the physician has an obligation to initiate CPR when *medically indicated*."[1] The report relies on the concept of a procedure's being "medically indicated."

Federal regulations have been established in the United States to protect seriously afflicted newborns from unwarranted refusal of treatment. These so-called Baby Doe regulations require that states have in place programs to respond to reports of medical neglect "including instances of withholding of *medically indicated* treatment from disabled infants with life-threatening conditions."[2] Once again, major life-and-death judgments rely on the concept of a procedure being medically indicated.

The critical issue, of course, is what is meant by *medically indicated.* Pharmacology textbooks list medical indications. Package inserts list conditions for which various medications are "indicated." But neither the regulation writers nor their critics have ever really asked what it means for a treatment or procedure to be "medically indicated."

The dictionary defines *indicate* as "to demonstrate or suggest the necessity or advisability of." To say that a procedure is "medically" indicated apparently would mean that medical science or medical people have demonstrated or suggested its necessity or advisability. The nature of that demonstration, the kind of evidence that medical professionals would bring forth, is not at all clear.

The Meaning of "Medically Indicated"

"MEDICALLY INDICATED" AS A
MATTER OF FACT

It is widely assumed among medical professionals that whether a treatment is indicated is, somehow, a matter of medical fact. If a drug produces no imaginable benefits for a particular diagnosis, it seems to be a matter of medical fact that that medication is not indicated. On the other hand, medications or other treatment interventions that produce clearly desirable effects are said to be indicated. It all seems so factual.

Yet judgments about the desirability of a predicted result can never be matters of fact, as we normally use the term. Such a judgment always involves values. Sometimes those value judgments are obvious and uncontroversial. But often they are not. For example, penicillin is said to be indicated for pneumonia (assuming that no *contraindications* are present, such as a history of anaphylaxis). But even in this apparently simple matter, it is not obvious that the result of overcoming a pneumococcal infection is always desirable. More than just religious objectors to the use of drugs might conclude that on balance, killing the microorganisms through the use of a chemotherapeutic agent is not desirable. Some patients with painful terminal illnesses and short life expectancies might well conclude that taking penicillin for pneumonia might prolong their agony and delay the inevitable. In fact, it is an evaluative judgment to conclude that it is desirable to prevent death from pneumonia, even when the survivor can live a long, healthy, happy life. It is an evaluative judgment about which there is a substantial consensus, but an evaluative judgment nevertheless. It is a judgment that long, happy life is better than death, which is an evaluation, not a matter of fact.

What is the role of medical science and medical expertise in making these evaluative judgments? Modern science routinely relies on a fact/value dichotomy.[3] Science can tell us the expected outcomes of alternative interventions and the probabilities of each possible outcome. It can tell us, for example, the probability of surviving a pneumococcal infection with and without penicillin of a particular dosage. It can predict the possibilities of various so-called side effects. What it cannot tell us is whether the possible outcomes are good or bad.

Some people hold that the evaluation of outcomes is purely subjective, that "value judgments" imply that there is no objective basis for deciding whether an outcome is good or bad. One need not take the subjective position regarding all evaluations, however. It is sometimes held that certain evaluative judgments—such as ethical evaluative judgments—have some objective basis. They are grounded in natural law, in religious decree, or in reason, which has an objective foundation.

Fortunately, it is not necessary to reach agreement on whether evaluative judgments are subjective or objective. Holders of either position ought to agree that the evaluations are not derivable directly from medical science. Regardless of whether it might be objectively good to preserve life of a particular form or only subjectively good, it cannot be determined from medical science alone that it is good to do so.

"MEDICALLY INDICATED" AS A MATTER OF PROFESSIONAL EVALUATION

The only reasonable conclusion is that deciding whether a treatment or procedure is good or bad is necessarily a matter of evaluation and cannot be determined directly from medical facts. Then what is the role of medical professionals in making such judgments? A somewhat more sophisticated account of what it means for a drug, treatment, or procedure to be medically indicated concedes that evaluation must take place, but then insists that these value judgments require medical professional competence.

The most important version of this position holds that medical professionals become experts not only on a set of facts and a scientific method, but also on a set of values, sometimes called medical values. These values, it is held, are inherent in a practice or profession.[4] They are inherent in what it means to be a physician. They are learned during the long process of socialization in medical school and the apprenticeship system to which young physicians are exposed. According to these analyses, the goal of medicine is to preserve or restore health. Edmund Pellegrino, a physician/philosopher who is the chairman of the President's Council on Bioethics, claims that just by understanding what medicine is one can figure out that the goal or "end" of a professional in the field must be to promote the health of the patient and that any behavior that is not undertaken for this purpose is not part of the physician's inherent mission. These values, which are supposedly absorbed in professional education, include the importance of prolonging life, relieving suffering, promoting health, and so forth. These claims have bite because many things that doctors might do are not, according to Pellegrino and other defenders of this notion, designed to promote health. Some things that are not inherent in the goal of promoting health might include physician participation in questioning military prisoners, executing criminals using medical means, and rationing health care to increase insurance company profits. Although many people might criticize these uses of medicine, there are other uses of medical skills not designed to promote health that many might see as more defensible, such as cosmetic surgery, birth control, and forensic medicine in criminal investigations.

Assume, for purposes of discussion, that physicians really do learn some set of professional values in their education and that these form the basis of clinical judgments about which interventions are "medically indicated." If so, then a statement that a procedure is "medically indicated" means merely that medical people have assessed the probable benefits and harms of its use in a particular circumstance and have found that, based on these special professional values, the net benefits are greater than those of any alternative course of action. If this is what it means for a drug or other medical procedure to be medically indicated, it creates two insurmountable problems.

Value Conflicts Internal to Medical Professionalism

First, as we saw in chapter 3, assuming that medical professionals make assessments based on a set of "medical values," there is not just one medical good; there are several medical goods, and sometimes they will conflict with one another. Any reasonable statement of the goals of medicine will contain multiple objectives that sometimes conflict: preserving life and relieving suffering, for example. In order to determine that a drug is medically indicated for a particular condition, one must determine not only that it will preserve life or relieve suffering, but that it will offer the proper mix of these goals.

In recent medical history there was a deviant interpretation of the goal of medicine that gave a first and absolute priority to preserving life. That was never the position of classical Hippocratic medicine. It has been established that the duty to preserve life is, in fact, a duty without classical roots.[5] It has never been endorsed by any formal medical professional association. To be sure, it is an accepted ethical position of some religious groups, such as Orthodox Jews. It is—and should be—respected, but as a religious ethical conclusion, not a consensus of medical professionals about what is inherent in the practice of medicine. Even many Hippocratic physicians didn't buy into this priority.

The problem is that if judgments about when interventions are medically indicated are to be based on the values internal to the practice of medicine, then the medical profession as a whole must be able to balance these and other apparently competing values properly. We must be told not only that it is inherent in medicine to preserve life and relieve suffering, but also exactly when it is appropriate to sacrifice life preservation in order to prevent suffering, and vice versa. There is absolutely no reason to assume that physicians, as a professional group, do or should agree on these value trade-offs. Health professionals, like all other persons, vary in their judgments about the balancing of competing values and goals. The task of reaching agreement about the proper balance seems both impossibly difficult and pointless.

Value Conflicts between Professional Medicine and Other Value Systems

Even if the medical profession could somehow magically reach a consensus on the proper balance between preserving life and relieving suffering, that still wouldn't settle the matter. Different patients with different beliefs and values may favor a different balance. Orthodox Jews and Jack Kevorkian don't see the question in the same way, and there is no need for them to. Some uses of medical interventions probably are so offensive they should be banned. Using drugs to kill your estranged spouse is not nice. It should be illegal. That is not because doctors have all agreed killing your ex is immoral; it is because society has concluded that doing so is so wrong that it must be banned. In the end it really doesn't matter what physicians think. It doesn't even matter what the medical profession as a whole thinks. It is a value question. On value questions the individual, including the individual layperson, has standing to form an opinion. If the consensus is that the behavior is so bad that it cannot be tolerated in a civil society, then society can and should ban it. Otherwise, a liberal society will try to tolerate individual value judgments, especially when acting on those judgments doesn't harm others. It can't be up to the medical profession to decide when face-lifts or abortions or murder of one's wife is unacceptable. In most cases, individual doctors should have the same rights of conscience as everyone else. No doctor, for example, should be required to perform an abortion if doing so violates his or her conscience, but that doesn't mean that either a woman's gynecologist or the professional association of gynecologists should have the authority to make the value judgment about whether an abortion is right for her. For the same reasons, your doctor cannot judge when to remove a cast from a broken arm or when to take statin drugs to lower cholesterol based on the values that he or his profession happens to hold.

Even if we could get the entire profession to agree that one particular mix of values internal to medicine is the correct one, there is no reason to accept the idea that that set of values is appropriate for persons who are not members of that professional community. Those persons would instead derive their own values from other sources—from religious, philosophical, and ethical traditions outside professional medicine. In fact, it is reasonable to suppose that special values about life preservation and relief of suffering lead people to choose medicine as a career in the first place. If so, we should expect that the value consensus reached by such people would be different from that of the general population. Medical professionals can be expected to hold different values and therefore can be expected to get the wrong answer in deciding for patients when treatments are worthwhile.

This is especially true when we realize that decisions about medical treatments will reasonably take into account a much wider range of value concerns than merely those on the medical professional's agenda. Reasonable laypeople will want to consider not only life preservation, relief of suffering, promotion of health, and the like, but also economic costs, the impact on one's family, the long-term ecological concerns, and just plain matters of taste. In other words, even if some constellation of medical values would be served by an intervention, other concerns may rule it out.

One possible interpretation is that an intervention is "medically indicated" if it is in accord with the value consensus of medical professionals (even though it is unreasonable to expect laypeople to share that value consensus). Another would be that an intervention is "medically indicated" if it corresponds with a layperson's medical agenda, while recognizing that any reasonable layperson will have an agenda that extends well beyond the medical. In either interpretation, claiming that a procedure is medically indicated says very little about what a reasonable person ought to do when all things are considered.

The Implications: Two Examples

The implications of all of this are radical. The new medicine undercuts the widespread assumption that deciding whether an intervention is medically indicated is a decision based on science or on the objective medical judgments of competent professionals. Consider two examples: the use of the concept "medically indicated" in pharmacology and related clinical sciences, and its use in public policy discourse.

"MEDICALLY INDICATED" IN PHARMACOLOGY

The idea of a drug being "medically indicated" is common in pharmacology (the scientific study of the actions of drugs). A similar notion is used in surgery, internal medicine, and other clinical sciences in referring to procedures and interventions thought to be beneficial on balance. In pharmacology, an author of an article or a textbook often claims that a drug is medically indicated for certain conditions. Normally, this assertion is accompanied by a list of conditions for which the drug is "contraindicated." It appears that these are claims rooted only in good medical science, but that appearance is deceptive.

For an author to claim that a drug is indicated is to say that according to someone's values, the medical or total benefits of the drug exceed the harms from the drug, taking into account the condition being discussed. Insofar as a pharmacologist is making claims about total benefits, she is clearly beyond her sphere of expertise. Such a judgment would require comparing the total benefits of the drug with the total negative consequences. This takes the pharmacologist into the realm of economic, religious, social, and aesthetic trade-offs, in which she clearly has no special competence.

Even if the judgment is limited to medical benefits, however, the claim is problematic. Consider, for example, the assertion that a particular non-narcotic analgesic, such as ibuprofen or acetaminophen, is indicated for the pain of a headache. Underlying this claim are some obvious evaluative judgments, such as that it is bad to have a headache, but also some subtler ones. For example, it might include the judgment that the benefit of eliminating the headache outweighs the one-in-ten-thousand or one-in-a-hundred-thousand risk of a particular blood problem (called a *dyscrasia*) that could result from the use of the drug. That judgment is extremely difficult to make, even for someone limiting her attention to so-called medical values. It depends not only on how bad it is to risk the blood dyscrasia, but also on how bad it is to have a headache. There is simply nothing in a doctor's training that gives him or her any authority to decide how to compare the harm of a headache with the harm of the blood dyscrasia. The television commercials tell us over and over to "ask your doctor," but asking your doctor is nothing more than asking the expert on the body for his or her religious, philosophical, or cultural preferences about taking a very small risk of a serious problem in order to have a good chance of relieving a relatively minor one. Medical school can't teach doctors the right answer to that kind of question.

"MEDICALLY INDICATED" IN PUBLIC POLICY

A similar problem emerges in public policy. Often in debates over insurance, research procedures, the right of access to care, FDA labeling, or the limits of treatment refusal by patients and their surrogates, policy makers make use of the concept of medical indication. Insurance will cover medically indicated treatments, community health clinics will provide indigents with the care that is medically indicated, and parents will be permitted to refuse treatment only when it is not medically indicated.

These are all sneaky attempts to convert the evaluative judgment into a scientific judgment. They make it appear as though medical science by itself can determine when a treatment is appropriate and when it is not. A governor debating funding of medication for AIDS patients was quoted as saying he did not oppose care that was medically indicated. A catastrophic health insurance plan provided that generic drugs should be dispensed except when trade name products were medically indicated. In a DNR (do not resuscitate) protocol, physicians are permitted to override familial treatment-refusal decisions when resuscitation was medically indicated. If you are confused by these policies, you should be. They are all attempts to convince us that someone's value judgments are objective and derived from medical science.

CASE 8.1

The Baby Doe Regulations and Medical Indications

Consider the Baby Doe regulations of the 1980s, regulations that to this day govern when parents are permitted to refuse life support for their infants. Those regulations say that it is medical neglect to withhold "medically indicated" treatment from a disabled infant with a life-threatening condition, to fail to provide "treatment (including appropriate nutrition, hydration, and medication) which, in the treatment physician's (or physicians') reasonable medical judgment, will be most likely to be effective in ameliorating or correcting all such conditions."[6] "Medically indicated" is made to sound like a judgment based on medical science. However, it relies on the clinician's "reasonable medical judgment" that the intervention is likely to be effective in "ameliorating or correcting" the conditions. Both *ameliorating* and *correcting* are evaluative judgments with considerable ambiguity.

The regulations appear to be requiring treatment when it will save a baby's life. The regulation writers are trying to leave to medical judgment only the determination of whether an intervention will increase the chances of survival. Even that position requires a normative judgment—that treatment should always be rendered whenever it will preserve life. That is a determination that policy makers have a right to make. It adds nothing, however, to call all such treatments "medically indicated." If the regulation writers believed that baby's lives should always be preserved whenever it was possible to do so, they really ought to say so. Calling these treatments "medically indicated" only says that, based on our value judgments, these are appropriate interventions. An ethical evaluation has been couched in language making it sound scientific.

That the regulation writers are making a value judgment is further revealed by the fact that three exceptions to the requirement of providing life-prolonging treatment are given. According to the writers, the term "medically indicated" does not include treatment that would merely prolong dying, treatment of the infant who is irreversibly comatose, or treatment that is virtually futile and inhumane. There is absolutely nothing, aside from ethical judgments, that makes treatment under these conditions any less medically indicated; in all three instances it would prolong infants' lives. There may be good moral reasons why treatment ought not be provided in these circumstances: It is merely temporarily life prolonging in the case of the inevitably dying infant, it is deemed of no value in the case of the comatose infant, and it is inhumanely burdensome in the case of care that is virtually futile. Many moral systems recognize that it is not morally required to offer treatment in such circumstances, but there is absolutely no reason to say in these situations that treatment is "medically not indicated." It is just a fancy way of saying that the writers don't think it is of any value.

The Baby Doe regulations may or may not be ethically sound. There are instances in which someone might decide a treatment is morally expendable even though none of the three conditions of the Baby Doe regulations is met. For example, Catholic moral theology holds that treatment is morally expendable if it is gravely burdensome even though it is not virtually futile. An Orthodox Jew or a federal regulation writer who disagrees has every right to do so, based on his or her religious or philosophical system of values, but it is meaningless to call treatment in such circumstances "medically indicated." That is simply an effort to cast as scientific necessity what is actually an ethical judgment.

The regulations provide one further example in their definition of "medically indicated" of an attempt to medicalize what are essentially evaluative judgments. The regulations specify that "appropriate" nutrition, hydration, and medication are medically indicated even in cases in which no further treatment is necessary. The withholding of such nutrition, hydration, and medication is considered the withholding of a medically indicated treatment. But in what sense are these medically indicated?

It is possible to adopt an ethical position that nutrition, hydration, and medication are morally required even for infants for whom a decision has been made that no other treatment should be provided. That is not a very plausible position. It is not the position of the AMA, American law, the Catholic Church, or any other religious group. If someone wanted to take that position, he or she would have the right to do so. It adds nothing, however, to call such treatment medically indicated. It is simply morally required according to holders of this view.

To make matters more complicated, according to the Baby Doe regulations, only "appropriate" nutrition, hydration, and medication are medically indicated. Presumably, the authors had in mind excluding the feeding of an infant with a tracheoesophageal fistula (an opening between the windpipe and the tube where food should pass) when oral feeding would actually cause the infant's death. However, deciding that it is appropriate to feed other infants for whom other treatment is being withheld is, once again, a value judgment that has nothing to do with medical science. There is an emerging consensus that any nutrition can be viewed as useless or burdensome when it merely prolongs the dying process of a comatose or suffering semiconscious patient. The writers of the Baby Doe regulations realize that government regulations do not normally announce value judgments particularly in controversial areas, that it would be nicer to dress them up as scientific. To do so, they claim that the treatments they believe should be provided are "medically indicated" whereas those that do not square with their values are not indicated.

Although there are also opinions and state laws to the contrary, the crucial point is that whether nutrition and hydration are ever expendable is a matter of ethical and other value judgment, not medical fact. That is why reasonable people might so understandably disagree on such issues.

To say that an intervention is indicated is to say that someone has made an assessment and found that based on his or her values and beliefs, the treatment is worth pursuing. If calling something medically indicated is just a subtle way of saying it is desired based on a particular set of values, then what is the implication for the relation of the medical profession, the government, and the general population in making such decisions? It appears to medicalize crucial ethical and policy determinations and to transfer decision-making power from public officials and laypersons to those with medical expertise.

Because calling something medically indicated is a matter of value judgment and not medical fact, it is understandable for reasonable people to disagree on at least some such assessments. It is for this reason that at least in a liberal society, government regulation makes sense only in cases in which the value judgments made are so powerful and so convincing that they can be imposed on a dissenting minority. Surely that is sometimes the case, at least in decisions involving surrogates for incompetent patients. Parents are not permitted to abuse their children. The government has a legitimate role in preventing what is clearly child abuse. But, as I shall argue in chapter 13, it should permit some latitude in judgments about what constitutes abuse. Determining what that latitude should be is necessarily a nonscientific question. Referring to treatments as "medically indicated" simply hides the true nature of the choices being made, and it transfers critical policy questions to medical professionals who may not share the broader public's ethical and policy framework.

Because in the Baby Doe regulations example we are debating the wisdom or correctness of a value judgment and not a matter of medical fact, it is odd that the standard for deciding what would constitute an unacceptable result is, as the regulations specify, "the physician's reasonable medical judgment." It is not clear what is "medical" about the judgment that a particular kind of nutrition is required or expendable for a comatose infant. If the problem were one requiring medical knowledge, skill, or wisdom—the sort of question that at first appears at stake when one speaks of "medical indications"—then it would make sense for the physician's judgment to be the standard of reference. But if the issue of whether a treatment is indicated really comes down to the question of whether it is ethically appropriate, then it is hard to see why individual laypersons are not capable of making such choices, constrained, if necessary, by society to protect innocent life.

Deciding that an intervention is indicated is really deciding that it fits some set of beliefs and values. If the layperson's beliefs and values do not have intolerable impacts on others, then it is the layperson's call. Physicians should be permitted to cooperate in the plan of care chosen. Government should intervene only when there is a strong possibility of harm to unconsenting parties. Calling treatments that are judged overwhelmingly beneficial "medically indicated treatments" adds very little except confusion.

NINE

"Treatments of Choice" and "Medical Necessity"

Who Is Fooling Whom?

Closely related to the idea of a treatment being "medically indicated" are the concepts of "treatment of choice" and "medical necessity." If "medical indications" is a term that bootlegs value judgments, talking about "treatment of choice" and "medical necessity" is a major moonshining industry. The two expressions are closely related. "Treatment of choice" is the simpler, so let's attack there first.

"Treatments of Choice": Medicine Can't Make Choices for Us

Claiming that a particular drug is the drug of choice is simply to say that according to the values of the one making the claim, its benefit-harm ratio is better than that of any alternative for the same condition. If deciding that a drug is indicated is a necessarily evaluative process, deciding that it is better than alternatives is an even subtler evaluation, about which pharmacologists have no particular authority.

The Cardiac Arrhythmia

A 50-year-old patient is diagnosed as having cardiac arrhythmia. It involves premature ventricular contractions (PVCs), a rapid, irregular spontaneous contraction of the lower (ventricular) chambers of the heart. Even though the patient feels no symptoms, there are over 600 irregular beats an hour. If the irregular electrical firings continue, there could be a fatal fibrillation. There is a wide range of plausible treatment options.

There are four classes of medications on the market to suppress the arrhythmias (membrane-stabilizing agents, beta-blockers, repolarization inhibitors, and calcium channel blockers). Some of the classes have subclasses. Although they all suppress the irregular heart rhythm, there is no definitive evidence that suppressing them lowers the mortality risk. In each class of agents, there are many different drugs, each with slightly different desired effects and side effects. There are many different dosage levels and routes of administration—short acting, long acting, and so forth. There are different manufacturers, different costs, and different risk profiles involved. Some clinicians are sufficiently concerned about the side effects that they recommend to their patients that no medication be used. Other clinicians use modest pharmacological intervention with low risk and proportionally low suppression of the arrhythmias. Others more aggressively suppress the PVCs, believing that, on balance, more good is done. The choices involve matters that are not trivial. The side effects range from nausea, vomiting, diarrhea, headache, and ringing in the ears, to unwanted changes in heart rhythm, a lupus erythematosus-like syndrome, coma, and even death. The dose forms range from a simple, one-a-day capsule to more complex combinations, taking different medications on different several-times-a-day schedules. The costs range from nothing to several hundred dollars a year for the rest of the patient's life. There are easily over a hundred possible courses of action, each of which has its own unique combination of advantages and disadvantages and might be favored depending on the patient's idiosyncratic circumstances and values and what one considers to be the correct theory of the good.

A naive patient's arrhythmia will be discovered by a physician who will assess the options and recommend either no medication or some variant of conservative or more aggressive medication. That physician will opt for one (or more) of the classes of drugs, some route of administration, dose range, cost, and profile of side effects and will write the prescription, subject, whether the patient realizes it or not, to the consent of the patient. Perhaps the physician will discuss with the patient some of the variables of the decision and will give the patient a chance to object.

Several drugs are available. Examples include propafenone (Rythmol), amiodarone (Cordarone, Pacerone), disopyramide (Norpace), dofetilide (Tikosyn), sotalol (Betapace), procainamide (Procanbid, Promine, Pronestyl), flecainide (Tambocor), and quinidine (Quinidex Extentabs, Quinaglute), as well as beta-blockers or calcium channel blockers. Each drug has its own mechanisms of action and a unique package of side effects. Not only do the drugs affect people differently, but people experiencing the same effects may evaluate those effects differently. Slight dizziness may be a trivial annoyance for one person, but a major problem for others. Each drug comes in various dose levels. Many can be administered in various ways: tablets, capsules, liquid form, or injection. To claim that one package of benefits and harms is the best—is the treatment of choice—is silly.

Not only do different drugs make the list of treatment options for different people, they may get ranked differently based on idiosyncratic preferences and concerns of each patient. For a textbook writer to claim one drug is the treatment of choice shows the chutzpah of the medical scientist.

"Medical Necessity": The Absurdity of the "Note from the Doctor"

One final term makes our list of words that make no sense in the world of postmodern medicine. The term "medical necessity" has surfaced from time to time to convey that someone has made a judgment that a procedure or a behavior is so important that no one could choose to reject it.

The term had a prominent place in the abortion literature of the 1960s in the era before *Roe v. Wade* when women could get certified to have abortions only if they could convince some physician to attest that the procedure was medically necessary.

No abortion is ever medically necessary—provided a woman is willing to pay the price of forgoing the abortion, which might be steep, even death. If the price is death, for most of us that would be a strange choice. No matter how tragic an abortion is, almost everyone recognizes that in rare cases aborting is important to save the life of the woman. Nevertheless, some women find abortion so abhorrent that they are willing to risk even death to avoid the procedure.

CASE 9.2

Birth at Any Price

I recall one woman in a clinic who was so militantly committed to a pregnancy and placed such high value on the life of her unborn child that she chose to continue the pregnancy even though her doctors warned her it seriously jeopardized her life. She had already experienced three times the life-threatening event of a ruptured uterus. Doctors told her it was going to happen again. Even the conservative Catholic doctor admitted that, even though the Church would not support it, this was that rare case in which the life of the mother forced him to recommend that she abort the pregnancy. For the doctor, continuing the pregnancy was just too dangerous. The priest who was involved was even willing to accept the reality. He refused to counsel her against the abortion.

But this courageous, feisty woman saw it differently. Even at the risk of her own life, she wanted to give that baby a chance. For her it was the right choice. She talked them into maintaining the pregnancy long enough for her to deliver by Caesarian at 30 weeks, when the fetus had matured to the point that the doctors thought it had a fighting chance.

She knew exactly what she was doing. She insisted that her pregnancy would continue. She would risk her own life. For her, the healthcare team's job was to keep that paper-thin part of her uterus from tearing as long as possible. It is not the decision I would ever have made, but it was right for her. No medical science can prove her wrong.

This woman's position might not have been the one most people would have taken. Even her antiabortion doctors were shocked. But there is nothing wrong with her choice, provided she understood the risks and held the values she held. To do anything else would have been irrational. Nothing makes that abortion "medically necessary."

On the other hand, some moderates on abortion compare those abortions thought of as being necessitated by the life or serious health concerns with so-called "elective abortions." If you stop and think about it, that language makes no sense either. In a free country all abortions are elective. None is compulsory. What people have in mind when they refer to elective abortion is abortion for social, economic, or psychological reasons. The reasoning seems to be that these reasons are less weighty so women would not be forced to abort. By contrast, abortion to save the life of the woman seems compelling. One would think that the opposite of "elective" would be "compulsory," but the term "therapeutic" is used. It is as if the relief from ending a pregnancy for critical psychological or social reasons couldn't count as therapy.

Even if a procedure is proposed to achieve some medical benefit, it is not a necessary procedure; even if it is proposed for nonmedical reasons, the procedure may still be critically important in the life interests of the patient. In neither case, however, is the procedure medically necessary.

Physician involvement in certifying medical necessity for abortion suggests a more pervasive problem. Doctors have, for decades, been called into service to justify or excuse behaviors that are otherwise intolerable. Doctors can classify persons as mentally ill and thus exempt them from many norms of adult behavior. They can provide the critical authorization for insurance companies to pay for health professional services. They can get people excused from school or work.

Often this excusing comes in the form of a "note from the doctor." In school, children can get authorizations to miss class, take drugs in school, avoid eating cafeteria food, and participate in contact sports by having the precious written statement from the authority figure that commands attention—the doctor. The logic behind such note writing was presumably that people who were sick or disabled had a legitimate right to be exempt from certain requirements. Alternatively, a certification that one was not ill or disabled was sufficient to permit participation in strenuous or risky physical activities. Similarly, employees—especially low-status employees—could be excused from their work responsibilities by producing a written statement from their doctors.

The critical problem, however, is that merely being certified as ill or disabled cannot automatically lead to a policy judgment that the individual is exempt from social responsibility. A child who particularly disliked a required swimming class was able to persuade his parents to get a note from their pediatrician indicating that ear infections and a poorly functioning labyrinth of the ear caused balance problems when the child got water in his ear.

There was some truth to the claim that the child suffered from a balance problem that was made worse by ear infections, which might have been related to swimming. The excusing of the child from the class, however, involved a much more complex set of issues. Setting aside the question of whether it is the responsibility of the school to force all children into swimming class, if such a decision is made, it must rest on an abstract judgment that swimming has lifesaving value, is good recreation, or builds character. The real issue is whether the burdens to the child caused by ear problems provided enough of a rationale to offset those purported benefits from compulsory swimming class. The physician, who, at most, can claim expertise on whether the ear problems were related to swimming, was in no position to make the decision that these social goods should be overridden by the medical problems.

Similarly, physicians are not in a good position to decide whether an employee's medical condition justifies an exemption from responsibilities at the workplace. That judgment would necessarily require considering how important it is for the employee to do the work, how disruptive it would be for a medically disabled employee to be on the job, and whether there are fellow employees who can cover for the employee who is excused. It is hardly a set of issues about which a physician can make an informed decision. The doctor's note is, at most, a certification of a patient's medical problems, not a justified excuse from responsibility. That would take the judgment of someone who has a much broader perspective.

The terminology of the new medicine will have to be different from the talk of doctor's orders, treatments of choice, and medical necessity. Any major change in a social institution requires the creation of a new language. Adult females can't be called "girls" any longer. People with mental impairment cannot be called "imbeciles" or "morons." Obese people are seldom called "fat" anymore (but we shall see in chapter 14 that some prefer being called "fat" to hearing the medicalized, but still judgmental, euphemism "overweight").

In the new medicine, doctors won't give "orders." They may educate, make suggestions, or give advice, but they will not order people to follow procedures. They won't "discharge" patients from hospitals. Textbooks won't be able to claim that certain treatments are "medically indicated" or that certain ones are so good that they are "treatments of choice." No procedure— even a lifesaving one—will be "medically necessary."

Finding replacement terms may not always be easy. "Mentally retarded" replaced more harsh-sounding terms, only to take on its own stigma and be replaced with the currently fashionable "persons with intellectual disability." One term that seemed to signal a transition to the new medicine was "informed consent." In the next chapter we will see that it may not be around too long. It may be only what could be called a transition terminology.

II

NEW CONCEPTS FOR THE NEW MEDICINE

TEN | Abandoning Informed Consent

Consent emerged as a concept central to the late stages of modern medical ethics. Often the term is used with a modifier, such as *informed* or *voluntary* or *full*, and is loosely used in phrases like "fully informed and voluntary consent." Modern ethics in health care could hardly function without the notion of consent.

Although we might occasionally encounter an old-guard, retrograde longing for the day when physicians did not have to go through the process of obtaining consent, the necessity of consent is now taken as a given, at least at the level of theory. To be sure, we know that actual consent is not obtained in all cases, and even when consent is obtained, it may not be adequately informed or autonomous. For purposes of this discussion, I shall not worry about the deviations from the ideal; rather, the focus will be on whether consent ought to be the goal. In this chapter I will argue that in the world of the new medicine, consent won't cut it.

This consensus in favor of consent may turn out to be all too facile. "Consent" may be a "transition concept," one that appears on the scene as an apparently progressive innovation, but after a period of experience turns out to be only useful as a transition to a more thoroughly revolutionary concept.[1]

The thesis of this chapter is that consent is merely a transitional concept. Although it emerged in the field as a liberal, innovative idea, its time may have passed, and newer, more enlightened formulations may be needed.

Consent means approval of or agreement with the actions or opinions of another; terms such as *acquiescence* and *condoning* appear in the dictionary definitions. In medicine, the physician or other health-care provider will, after reviewing the facts of the case and attempting to determine what is in the best interest of the patient, propose a course of action for the patient's concurrence. A few decades ago it might have been considered both radical and innovative to seek the patient's acquiescence in the professional's clinical judgment; by now that may not be nearly enough.

I have argued in this book that there no longer exists any basis for presuming that the clinician can even guess at what is in the overall best interest of the patient. If that is true, then a model in which the clinician decides on what he or she believes is best for the patient, pausing only to elicit the patient's concurrence (consent), will no longer be sufficient. We increasingly will have to go beyond patient consent to a model in which plausible options are presented. Those options may be accompanied by the professional's recommendation regarding a personal preference among them (based on the professional's personally held beliefs and values), but no rational or "professional" basis will be found for even guessing at which one might be truly in the patient's best interest. In order to demonstrate that the concept of consent will no longer be adequate for the era of contemporary medicine, some work will be in order.

In this chapter, after summarizing the emergence of the consent doctrine, I will see what we can learn from what is called *axiology*—the philosophical study of the theory of the good. This will call into question the adequacy of *consent* as a means of legitimating clinical decisions. This, I suggest, will provide a basis for demonstrating why experts in an area such as medicine should not be expected to guess correctly what course is in the patient's interest and therefore should not be able to propose a course to which the patient's task is mere consent or refusal. That will set the stage for the next chapter, in which I will propose a postmodern alternative to patient consent.

The History of Consent

The notion of consent is a relatively recent phenomenon.[2] None of the classical documents in the ethics of professional medicine contained anything resembling a notion of consent—informed or not. Autonomy of decision making—especially lay decision making—was not in the operating framework. For example, neither the Hippocratic Oath nor any of the other Hippocratic writings say anything about consent or any other form of patient participation in decision making.[3] The Oath explicitly prohibits even disclosure of information to patients. Until the revision of 1980, the American Medical Association's *Current Opinions* did not include any notion of consent either. To this day the AMA *Opinions* permit physicians to treat without consent when the physician believes that consent would be "medically contraindicated."[4]

Consent is essentially a twentieth-century phenomenon, but one that has its roots in post-Reformation affirmation of the individual and the liberal political philosophy and related judicial system derived from it rather than in professional physician ethics.[5]

Although classical medical ethics had no doctrine of informed consent, modern medicine did begin making some room for the notion. Wide recognition of the importance of patient concurrence in a medical intervention first arose in research involving human subjects. The Nuremberg Code gives first-place prominence to the consent requirement.[6] In clinical medicine, explicit consent, at least until very recently, has been reserved for more controversial treatments and for choices that are perceived as "ethically exotic." Consent has often been invoked for treatment decisions in which the patient is seen as drawing on ethical and other values coming from outside of medicine. This arises more often in the refusal of consent than approval of treatment. For instance, patients now sometimes are given the opportunity to refuse consent for certain death-prolonging interventions during a terminal illness.

Sometimes the notion of consent notion gets a bit muddled—as when patients are asked to "consent" to DNR (do not resuscitate) orders. The idea of consenting to an "order" is strange, but the idea of consenting to nontreatment is even stranger. A more appropriate language would refer to refusal of consent to resuscitation rather than consenting to nonresuscitation. (When we choose medical treatment over surgery, we don't consent to nonsurgery.)

Modern medicine reluctantly has made room for the consent doctrine and has recognized, at least in theory, the right of patients to consent and refuse consent to certain kinds of treatment. Explicit consent usually is reserved for these more complex and exotic decisions. It is still common to hear people distinguish between treatments for which consent is required and those for which it is not. Surely, it would be better to speak of those for which consent must be explicit and others that still require consent even though the consent can be implied or presumed. For example, many people might say that routine blood drawings of modest amounts can be performed without consent. This would be more appropriately described as being done without explicit consent. No specific information needs to be transmitted. The mere extending of the arm should count as an adequate consent. Most patients know there will be a slight prick from the needle and probably even realize that there could be minor bruising. Some people drawing blood might mention the slight risk of infection, but that risk seems rather obvious and probably does not need explicit mention.

Likewise, when twentieth-century physicians wrote prescriptions, they were supposed to review the alternatives and choose the best medication; select a brand name or generic equivalent; and choose a route of administration, a dosage level, and length of use of the medication. The patient might have signaled "consent" simply by accepting the prescription and getting it filled at the local pharmacy.

Until now no one who accepts the general idea of consent has seriously questioned whether this approach—which permits explicit consent for special and complex treatment, including research and surgery, and implicit or presumed consent for more routine procedures—is adequate. In fact, the consent model buys into the traditional authoritarian understanding of clinical decision making more than many people realize. As in the days prior to the development of the consent doctrine, the clinician still is supposed to draw on his or her medical knowledge to determine what he or she believes is in the best interest of the patient and then propose that course of treatment. Terms such as "doctor's orders" may be in the process of being replaced by more appropriate images, but the physician is still expected to determine what is "medically indicated," the "treatment of choice," or what in his or her "clinical judgment" is best for the patient. The clinician then proposes that course, subject only to the patient's signal of approval (through either word or action) of the physician-determined plan.

Consent and the Theory of the Good

This pattern no longer makes sense. It still rests on the outdated presumption that the clinician's moral responsibility is to do what is best for the patient, according to his or her ability and judgment, and that there is some reason to hope that the clinician can determine what is in the patient's best interest.

EMERGING PROBLEMS WITH THE
CONCEPT OF BEST INTEREST

The idea in medical ethics of doing what is best for the patient has achieved the status of an unquestioned platitude, but, as we have seen in this volume, this platitude, like many platitudes, may not stand the test of more careful examination. On several levels the problems are beginning to surface. The implication is that there are many situations in which doctors should not do what they believe is best, even if they can figure out what that might be.

1. The Best-Interest Standard in Surrogate Decisions

The "best-interest standard" has become the standard for surrogate decision making in cases in which the wishes of the patient are unknown and substituted judgment based on the patient's beliefs and values is impossible. But the best-interest standard, if taken literally, is terribly implausible. In fact, no decision maker is held to it, in practice. Newly discovered problems show why doctors cannot merely do what they think is best.

a. Subjective Variation in Judgments

Two problems arise. First, since such judgments are terribly complex and subjective, it is now widely accepted that the surrogate need not choose literally what is best. It would be extremely difficult, if not impossible, to determine whether the absolute best choice has been made.

CASE 10.1

Why a Doctor Should Give a Boy a Quack Remedy

A doctor at one of the best hospitals in the country was confronted with a crisis. A two-year-old boy named Chad Green was suffering from leukemia for which the physician prescribed chemotherapy.[7] It had a fair chance of working. The problem was that his parents were members of an alternative lifestyle community that thought chemotherapy was too harsh. They wanted to treat their boy with a special diet of macrobiotic rice and a compound called Laetrile, which was an extract of apricot pits. Although there was no scientific evidence supporting this therapy for leukemia, they believed it was better.

The doctor didn't agree. He believed that the orthodox treatment was best for the boy. The doctor had the authority to get a court order permitting him to treat the boy against the parents' wishes. He actually did go to court, but he was a very wise doctor. He knew that the calculation of the benefits and the harms of the alternatives in this case was very complicated. The chemotherapy had only about a 50% chance of working. Moreover, it had troublesome side effects. It could even kill the boy (although that was not likely). On the other hand, the rice and apricot pits probably wouldn't help, but they wouldn't hurt either, as long as they were obtained from a safe and clean source.

The doctor eventually made a deal with the parents that the court was willing to accept. He would personally obtain the extract from the apricot pits and administer the compound to the boy along with the special rice diet, provided the parents agreed to permit him to administer the chemotherapy.

Many doctors were troubled by this compromise. The doctor was cooperating in providing what the medical community believed was a quack remedy. Some minimal risk existed that the boy would react negatively to the extract or the diet, which were considered otherwise useless. It was believed that doctors shouldn't cooperate in the use of fraudulent, quack remedies and shouldn't expose the boy to any additional risk, however small. On the other hand, the doctor knew the risks of using the court to force the parents to go along with a treatment that they found unacceptable. The deal was one that neither the doctors nor the parents thought best, but it was a wise compromise. The compromise was in the ballpark and, given the parents' strong feelings, was perfectly acceptable.

Neither doctors nor parents are required to do literally what is best for the child as long as they provide a reasonably acceptable approximation. Doctors, as it turns out, make such compromises all the time. The alternative would be to take parents and guardians to court whenever the surrogate for an incompetent patient chooses a course that appears a little off base. Surrogates must be within reason. They need not literally choose the best course or even what they believe is best.

Surely, the opinion of the attending physician cannot serve as a definitive standard. A privately appointed, ethics committee might be better, but still not definitive. If every surrogate decision were taken to court, we still would not have absolute assurance that the best choice had been made. We expect, tolerate, and even encourage a reasonable range of discretion. That is why it makes sense to replace the best-interest standard with a "standard of reasonableness" or what could be called a "reasonable interest standard."[8]

b. Conflicting Surrogate Duties

There is a second reason why the best-interest standard is inappropriate for surrogate decision makings and cannot provide a definitive basis on which doctors should act. Often, surrogates have legitimate moral obligations to people other than the patient. Parents, for example, are pledged to serve the welfare of their other children. When best interests conflict, it is logically impossible to fulfill the best-interest standard for more than one child at the same time. Surely, all that is expected is that they pursue a reasonable balance of the conflicting interests.

2. Problems with Best Interest in Clinician Judgments

Although problems with the best-interest standard in surrogate decisions are more immediately apparent, a more fundamental problem arises when clinicians are held to the best-interest standard in an ethic of patient care.

In order for a clinician to guess at what the best course for the patient is, three assumptions must be true regarding a theory of the good. As we saw in chapters 4–6, first, the clinician must be able to determine what will best serve the patient's medical or health interest and how to trade off health interests with other interests; second, the clinician must be able to determine how the patient should relate the pursuit of his or her best interest to other moral duties that happen to conflict with the patient's interest; and, third, the clinician must be able to determine how to resolve conflicts between the patient's interests and the interests of others. It is terribly implausible to expect a typical clinician to be able to perform just one of these tasks correctly, let alone all three of them. If the clinician cannot be expected to guess at what serves the well-being of the patient and determine when patient well-being should be subordinated to other moral requirements, then there is no way he or she can be expected to propose a course of treatment to which the patient would offer mere consent.

ALTERNATIVE THEORIES OF THE GOOD

In order to understand the limits on the clinician's ability to propose a course that will maximize patient well-being, we need to examine briefly current accounts of what counts as "the good." Axiology—the study of theories of the good or the valuable—is a field of normative philosophical ethics that is in considerable turmoil. Fortunately for our purposes, any plausible contemporary theory leads to the same radical conclusion: There is no reason to believe that a physician or any other expert in only one component of well-being should be able to determine what constitutes the good for another being.

Determining what it means to say something is in someone's best interest turns out to be a very difficult task. Establishing the proper criteria for determining that one course or another maximizes the good for an individual is even harder. One major philosophical contributor to this debate suggests that there are at least three major groups of answers to the question of what is in someone's best interest.[9]

The first approach holds that what best serves someone's interest is that which makes the person's life happiest. (These are called hedonistic theories.) There is no reason why a physician would know the answer to the question of what makes a patient happiest.

A second approach holds that what is best for someone is what would in one way or another fulfill his or her desires (recognizing that one's desires may include many ends other than happiness). (These are called desire-fulfillment theories.) There is no reason to assume that a clinician—a specialist in one relatively narrow aspect of well-being and a relative stranger to the patient—should be able to guess either at what would make the patient most happy or what would fulfill a patient's desires.

The third group of theories of the good is collectively referred to as objective list theories.[10] As summarized by Derek Parfit, "According to this theory, certain things are good or bad for people, whether or not these people would want to have the good things, or to avoid the bad things. The good things might include rational activity, the development of one's abilities, having children and being a good parent, knowledge, and the awareness of true beauty."[11] Other people's lists of objective goods may differ, but, as Bernard Gert has argued, there is a remarkable convergence on the items for the list, as long as the items are kept quite general.[12]

Most uses of the concept of best interests in health-care ethics seem to rely on some theory of objective goods. If a physician is expected to first determine what is in the patient's best interest and then present it to the patient for consent, there must be a presumption of a good that is, in some sense, objective and knowable by someone who is committed to pursuing the patient's welfare. When the standard of best interest is used by a court or a theorist dealing with surrogacy decisions for patients whose personal wants, desires, preferences, and beliefs are unknown, they are operating on some notion that the good of the patient is objective and external to the patient.

What is striking here is that even with objective list theories, an enormous gap exists between what it would require to know what is "objectively in a patient's interest" and what the usual clinician can be expected to know about the patient. For example, many objective list theories include, as the things that are good for people, features such as spiritual well-being, freedom, sense of accomplishment, and "deep personal relationships."[13] Holders of such objective list theories claim that these are good for people regardless of whether they make people happy and, in contradistinction to desire-fulfillment theories, regardless of whether the individual desires these or even knows they are possible.

Certainly, a physician is not usually in a good position to determine whether a medical intervention will contribute to the patient's sense of accomplishment or to that individual's "deep personal relations." If this is true even for an objective theory of the good, there will be no way for the health professional to know whether the patient's good is served with a medical intervention without asking the patient. To put it bluntly, the only way to know whether an intervention is good medicine is to ask the patient.

Our conclusion seems clear: Regardless of the theory of the good chosen, there is no reason to assume that the health professional can be expected to know what will promote the best interest of the patient. This conclusion seems clear on its face for hedonistic and desire-fulfillment theories of the good. It is less obvious, but equally true, for objective theories of the good.

ELEMENTS OF WELL-BEING

The problem can be made clearer by looking at what could be called the spheres, or elements, of well-being. Regardless of the theory of the good, we can better understand what promotes the good for persons by asking what elements contribute to one's well-being. Another way of putting it would be, if one has a limited amount of personal resources—time, money, energy, and materiel—in what areas ought they be invested in order to maximize well-being?

1. The Main Elements of Well-Being

Several elements of life can be identified. These would surely include some concern with medicine or what could be called one's organic well-being. Closely related, but distinct, is psychological well-being.

It would be a terrible distortion to assume that well-being involved only the organic and psychological. Reasonable people would devote considerable attention and resources to other elements, including social, legal, occupational, religious, aesthetic, and other components that together make up one's total well-being. The general scheme is represented in figure 10.1.

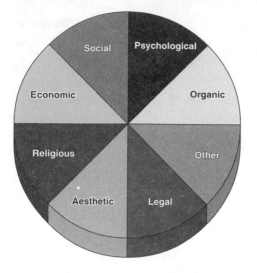

FIGURE 10.1
Elements of Spheres of
Well-being. (From Robert M.
Veatch, *Basics of Bioethics*,
Upper Saddle River, NJ:
Prentice-Hall, 2003, p. 52.)

There is no reason to assume that each slice of the pie should be the same size. By trading off emphasis on different slices, one should be able to increase or decrease the size of the total pie. Well-being is not a zero-sum game.

The problem is central to the concern about the concept of consent. It is unrealistic to expect experts in any one component (sphere) to be able to speak knowledgeably about well-being in the other components. Doctors are not experts on legal or spiritual well-being. Therefore, it makes no sense to expect them to devise proposed interventions that will promote the total well-being of the individual.

2. The Subcomponents of Organic or Medical Well-Being

One obvious response is to back off from the claim that the goal of medicine is to promote total well-being. A more modest formulation would be that the end of medicine is to promote not the total well-being of the patient, but the health—the medical good—of the patient. Although this is more realistic, it still creates two serious problems. First, even if the health professional were to limit concern to organic well-being, this component of well-being cannot be thought of as a single, univocal good. As we suggested in chapter 5, there are several, often competing, goods in the medical realm. Figure 10.2 shows that the organic well-being slice of the pie can be further subdivided into several more specific medical goods.

If a physician is to use "clinical judgment" to determine what will serve the medical good of the patient, he or she will have to possess a definitively

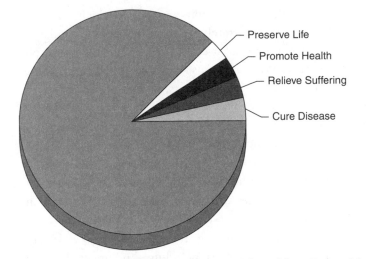

FIGURE 10.2 Elements of Medical Well-being. (Adapted from Robert M. Veatch, *The Basics of Bioethics*. Upper Saddle River, NJ: Prentice-Hall, 2003, p. 54.)

correct account of the relationship among these medical goods and how they should be traded off against one another. Unless someone is prepared to argue not only that there is a definitively correct relationship among these various medical goods, but also that the physician should be able to identify that relationship, even the more modest goal of recommending what is *medically* best for the patient will be illusory.

There is a second, more serious, problem with the strategy of expecting clinicians to recommend the medically best course and having the patient consent or refuse consent for that recommendation. At best, such a strategy will produce what is *medically* best for the patient. However, a realistic goal for a person is to maximize total well-being (subject to possible moral constraints requiring one to take into account the well-being of others and to act in ways that are morally required). Assuming that resources are not infinite, no rational person wants to maximize his or her health. Because less marginal benefit comes as greater amounts of resources are put into an area, it would be irrational to expect that one could maximize the size of the whole pie by maximizing the size of one of its pieces. Health professionals not only have to figure out how to balance the various medical goods against one another, they also have to realize that rational patients do not want that goal pursued, at least if it comes at the expense of goods in other spheres and lowers the patient's total well-being.

Recall the example in the previous chapter, in which a 40-year-old man is diagnosed as having moderately severe polyfocal ventricular arrhythmia consisting of PVCs at a rate of over 600 per hour. The typical physician in the era of consent would pick from scores of possible drugs, dosages, routes of administration, side effects, and costs, and then perhaps ask the patient to consent to the doctor's choice.

What the patient may not know is that another equally competent clinician with different instincts about how aggressive to be, which risks are worth taking, and what trade-offs with nonmedical well-being should be made will choose some other course and propose it for patient consent. Many of the possible choices that were rejected by this physician could be perceived as plausible by other responsible clinicians. The correct choice will depend on the trade-offs among the various medical goods and between the medical and nonmedical goods including a judgment about how the patient should spend marginal dollars. In such a situation, it is simply hubris for clinicians to believe that out of all these subtle value trade-offs to be made, they can come up with just the course that will maximize the patient's well-being.

Informed consent is a marvelous advance over the primitive paternalism of older medicine. It would at least give a patient a chance to reject the physician's proposed course. It remains, however, a relic of modern medicine, a minimal movement in the direction of recognizing the role of the active, responsible patient in his or her own medical decisions. If patients are ever to become active decision makers controlling their own health and healing based on their own beliefs and values, we will have to do better. Consent, the showpiece of modern medical ethics, will have to be abandoned.

ELEVEN

Why Physicians Get It Wrong and the Alternatives to Consent

Patient Choice and Deep Value Pairing

It should now be clear why it makes no sense to continue to rely on consent as the mode of transaction between professionals and their clients.

Why Physicians Should Guess Wrong

In order for a physician to estimate which treatment best serves the patient's interest, he or she first would have to develop a definitive theory of the relationship among various medical goods and pick the course that best serves the patient's medical good. Next, the clinician would have to estimate correctly the proper relationship between the patient's medical good and all other components of the good, so that the patient's overall well-being is served.

Even if this could be done, there is a final problem. In any decision, the well-being of the individual is only one element. Plausible consequentialist theories (such as utilitarianism) also insist that the good of other parties be taken into account. Plausible nonconsequentialist theories, including Kantian theories, natural law theories, much of Biblical ethics, and all other deontological theories, hold that knowing what will be in the best interests of persons does not necessarily settle the question of what the right thing to do is. Many patients may purposely consider options that do not maximize their well-being.

For one example, a patient may acknowledge that his well-being would be served if he lived longer but choose to sacrifice his interests to conserve resources for his offspring. For another example, a pregnant woman might conclude that her interests would be served if she had an abortion, but that such a course would still be morally wrong. Both of these people would rationally choose not to take the course of action that maximized their personal well-being. Even if physicians could figure out what maximizes medical well-being and how medical well-being should be related to other elements of well-being, that still does not necessarily lead to the course that is right. To know what is "good medicine" and what should be recommended for the patient's assessment and consent, one needs to know how to answer all three of these questions. There is no basis for assuming that physicians have any special expertise in answering any of them.

This may simply establish that physicians are no better than the rest of us at guessing what counts as the medical good, how the medical good relates to total good, and whether the patient's total good should be promoted. A defender of the emerging process of informed consent might respond by pointing out that physicians should at least be considered to be as good as any other layperson in answering these value theory questions. Because physicians clearly have technical expertise, if they are as good as anyone else at answering the value questions, would not efficiency lead to having the physicians combine the technical knowledge of the patient's case with their ordinary level of wisdom when it comes to making value judgments? This could lead to a recommended course of action for the patient. As long as the patient can decline, would that not be the most efficient way to maximize the patient's welfare?

There are two problems. First, this democratic theory of value that holds that professional experts are as good as others at guessing what maximizes the good can, at best, lead to a general estimate of what the typical person would consider to be good. If, however, any plausible value theory includes elements that are unique to the individual, then merely figuring out what would be good for the general person will not be good enough. We need to know what is good for this particular person. We need not hold to the liberal position that the individual is the best predictor of what serves his or her interest. All we need to acknowledge is that experts in a particular area are not the best at this task.

This leads to a second problem with relying on the claim that experts in one component of well-being should be as good as anyone else at determining the total good for the patient. Experts in any one component of well-being will answer the questions about what maximizes interests in an atypical fashion.

This is not because they are self-serving, trying to increase utilization of their services. I assume, perhaps naively, that most health professionals are altruistic and usually do a good job holding self-interest in check.

The problem is more theoretical and more fundamental. Anyone who has given his or her life to an area of professional specialization ought to be expected to value the contributions of that area in an atypical way. Cardiologists ought to believe atypically that cardiology does good for people. Presumably, that is one reason why people choose to enter a certain profession. Lawyers tend to think that the law helps people. Members of the clergy see particular value in spiritual goods. But this means that if they ask themselves what intervention will best promote the overall well-being of their client, they will give an answer that will be wrong in a systematic way. They will tend to provide the answer that would promote good outcomes as they understand the situation. Physicians predictably value the medical good differently from the way laypeople value it. They will overemphasize some elements of the medical good (such as preserving life) and underemphasize others (such as relieving suffering). They will give an answer different from that which a layperson, such as the patient, would give. They often, but not always, will overvalue the benefits of their field. Even if they undervalue those benefits, their evaluation is likely to be atypical.

Imagine one were to approach each professional group one by one and ask experts in each of the components of well-being in figure 10.1 what portion of an individual's total resources should be invested in their component. Then, if you were to sum the collective recommendations, it is likely that the total would exceed 100 percent of the available resources.

Experts not only make the value trade-offs atypically, they also make the moral trade-offs atypically. In short, if clinicians were asked to guess what will serve the best interest of the patient, they should be expected to come up with the wrong answer. Insofar as the consent process involves a clinician using personal judgment to guess what would be best for the patient, it still rests on the false assumption that clinicians can, at least tentatively, estimate what specific treatment interventions are in the individual patient's interests.

This should make it clear why relying on the consensus of medical experts does not provide an adequate way to figure out what the "treatment of choice" should be for the patient with the cardiac arrhythmia or any other medical treatment. One might hold the clinician to the "professional standard," choosing to recommend the drug that the majority of her colleagues similarly situated would have chosen. All that could do is tell us what people with the dominant value profile of the medical profession would choose under similar circumstances. It does not tell us what persons with the typical value profile of the average layperson would choose, let alone what one with the value profile of the specific patient would choose. As I will explain in chapter 24, the consensus of the profession does not provide an adequate basis for deciding what the "treatment of choice" is and what should be recommended to patients. The idea that a clinician can determine what is a "medically indicated" treatment for a patient rests on a confused understanding of what the skills of a physician can be expected to provide. If the clinician cannot be expected to figure out what is best for the patient, then he or she cannot obtain a valid consent to a recommended treatment of choice.

The Alternatives to Consent

If consent is inadequate as a mechanism for assuring that the patient's beliefs and values will shape that patient's medical decisions, then what are the alternatives?

CHOICE: THE LIBERAL ALTERNATIVE

Advocates of autonomy may prefer the concept of *choice* to that of *consent*. If "choice" is the approach, the patient would be presented with a list of plausible treatment options, together with a summary of the potential benefits and risks of each. It is important to emphasize that choice is conceptually different from consent and potentially could replace consent as the basis for patient involvement in health-care decisions.

This "liberal" solution, however, faces serious, probably insurmountable problems. First, if the choices that are plausible for the patient are contingent on the beliefs and values of the patient, then the professional cannot be sure that all of the plausible options are being presented unless he or she has the knowledge of the patient's beliefs and values that we have argued is normally unavailable. Second, some options—for example, suicide—may be so offensive to some practitioners that they ought not present them. Third, it is increasingly recognized that even the description of the "facts" necessarily must incorporate certain value judgments, such that even the good-willed clinician cannot give a value-free account of the likely outcomes of the alternatives. (This issue will be explored in detail in chapter 23.) In short, although the choice alternative may go partway toward giving the patient more active control, it is naive to believe it will be able to solve the problems with the consent model.

It should now be clear that the new medicine is more than just an appeal to patient autonomy. Autonomy is fine as an antidote to too much medical dominance. Consent and its partner, refusal of consent, provide the beginnings of a corrective, but in the end patients will not be able to take over every element of medical decision making. Doctors will, at minimum, have to provide the diagnosis and a summary of the treatment alternatives. Some of those alternatives may be so offensive to some doctors that they should not be required to even mention them, let alone recommend them. Something more than naked patient autonomy will be needed.

PAIRING BASED ON "DEEP VALUES"

There is another alternative worth considering. Although the typical clinician—even one who is skilled and passionately committed to maximizing the patient's welfare—cannot be expected to guess exactly what will be in the patient's best interest, there may be a special case in which there is reason to hope that the clinician's guess will come fairly close.

If the clinician knew the belief and value structure and socioeconomic and cultural position of the patient quite well, there would be some reason to hope for a good guess. Unfortunately, not only is that an ever-vanishing possibility, but even knowing the value system of the patient well probably would not be sufficient. The value choices that go into a judgment about what is best for someone else are so complex and subtle that merely knowing that person's values and trying to empathize will probably not be enough. There is ample evidence that unconscious value distortions will not only influence the clinician's judgment about what is best, but even influence the very interpretation of the scientific data. We will have more to say about this postmodern problem in chapter 23.

There might be more hope if the patient were to choose her cadre of well-being experts (lawyers, accountants, physicians, et al.) on the basis of what I will call their "deep" value systems. That way, when unconscious bias and distortion occur, as inevitably they must, they will tip the decision in the direction of the patient's own system.

I say "deep" value system because I want to make clear that I am not referring to a cursory assessment of the professional's personality, demeanor, and short-term tastes; that would hardly suffice. If, however, there were alignments—"value pairings"—based on the most fundamental worldviews of the layperson and professional, then there would be some hope. This probably would mean picking providers on the basis of their religious and/ or political affiliations, philosophical and social inclinations, and other deeply penetrating worldviews. To the extent that the provider and patient were of the same mind-set, then there is some reason that the technically competent clinician could guess fairly well what would serve the patient's interest—at least much of the time.

The difficulty in establishing a convergence of deep values cannot be underestimated. Surely, it would not be sufficient, for instance, to pair providers and patients on the basis of their institutional religious affiliations. Not all members of a religious denomination think alike. But there is reason to hope that people can find providers with similar deep value orientations, at least for certain types of medical services. For example, certain institutionalized health-care delivery systems are now organizing around identifiable value frameworks, recruiting professional and administrative staff on the basis of commitment to that value framework, and then announcing that framework to the public so as to attract only those patients who share the basic value commitment of the institution.

A hospice is organized around such a constellation of values. It recruits staff committed to those values and attracts patients who share that commitment. When hospice-based providers present options to patients, they should admit that they do not present all possible options. (They do not propose an aggressive oncology protocol, for instance; most would not present physician-assisted suicide or active mercy killing.) They should also admit that when they explain options and their potential benefits and harms, they do so in ways that incorporate a tone of voice or body language that reflects their value judgments. However, clients of a hospice (I'll argue in chapters 18 and 19 they shouldn't be called "patients") need be less concerned about this value encroachment than if they were discussing options with a provider who was deeply, instinctively committed to maximally aggressive life preservation. There will be biases, but they will be less corrupting of the layperson's own perspective.

Other delivery systems are beginning to organize around deep value orientations: Feminist health centers, holistic health clinics, and the National Institutes of Health Clinical Center all announce at least their general value orientations to potential patients.

Providing an institutional framework for pairing based on deep value convergence in more routine health care may be more difficult, but not impossible. HMOs could be organized by social and religious groups that could formally articulate certain value commitments. A Catholic HMO, like a Catholic hospital, could articulate to potential members not only a set of values pertaining to obstetrical and gynecological issues, but also a framework for deciding which treatments may be omitted because they are too burdensome. A liberal Protestant health-care system would announce a different framework; a libertarian secular system still another. A truly Protestant health-care system, for example, would probably reflect the belief that the layperson is capable of having control over the "text." The medical record, accordingly, would be placed in the patient's hands, just as the Bible was.

Such value pairings obviously will not match perfectly, but they should at least place provider and patient in the same general camp. Moreover, organizing health-care delivery on the basis of explicit value pairings would make both provider and patient aware that values are a necessary and essential part of health-care decision making, a part that cannot be avoided and cannot be handled adequately by merely obtaining the consent of the patient to a randomly assigned provider's guess about what would be best.

With such an arrangement, the problems that arise with use of consent for the normal random pairing of laypeople and professionals are mitigated. The clinician has a more plausible basis for guessing what would serve the interests of the patient and—more important—will let a system of beliefs and values influence presentation of medical information in a way that is more defensible. To be sure, such deep value pairing will not eliminate the problem of the necessary influence of beliefs and values on communication of medical facts, but it will structure the communication so that the inevitable influence will resemble the influence that the patient would have brought to the data, were he or she to become an authority on medical science.

Barring such radical adjustment in the basis for lay-professional pairings, there is no reason to believe that the process of consent will significantly advance the layperson's role in the medical decision-making process. The concept of consent will have to be replaced with a more radical, robust notion of active patient participation in the choice among plausible alternatives—either by getting much greater information to the patient or by actively selecting the professional on the basis of convergence of "deep" value systems.

| The End of Prescribing

Why Prescription Writing Is Irrational

In chapter 9 we discussed the foolishness of the note from the doctor. Yet, doctors write notes for their patients constantly. The law requires it for patients who want to get any of thousands of drugs. These drugs sometimes are called "legend" drugs. Even more outrageously, some manufacturers call them "ethical" drugs. The form the doctor signs is called a *prescription*.[1] It is a note to a pharmacist that is actually a legal document, an authorization for the pharmacist to dispense to the patient a drug that is otherwise, by federal law, illegal to possess. How did we get ourselves in the absurd position that mature adults in a free country cannot possess beneficial drugs for their own use unless they can find some physician someplace who will write them a note?

The physician who writes the note need not know the patient. He or she need not even have met the patient. He can prescribe over the telephone. In order to decide that the person desiring the medication is worthy of it, logic tells us that the physician ought to determine that the drug is good for the patient—that it is reasonably likely to do more good than harm. But, as we have been discovering, figuring out that a treatment will be beneficial for the patient is much harder than practitioners of modern medicine ever imagined. To prescribe a medication, the physician really should determine that it is the *best* available treatment—the *drug of choice*. This, however, is exactly what physicians cannot be expected to know about their patients.

To repeat our conclusion—to know what will benefit the patient, the physician will normally have to ask the patient. This means that before physicians write prescriptions authorizing patients to buy medications, they really should ask their patients what to write.

Confusions about Prescriptions

A closer look at the act of prescription writing reveals why this is so. For any typical medical problem, there is not just one possible treatment. There are both drug and nondrug options (including the option of watchful waiting). Even if the physician can correctly guess that a drug treatment fits the patient's values, many options still exist. There is often more than one drug available, each with its own risks and benefits, cost, and evidence of effectiveness. Not every patient with a medical condition will want to make the same risk-benefit trade-offs.

Even if the physician can correctly guess which chemical formula best fits the patient's values, he or she will still need to pick a dosage form. An injectable form will deliver an accurately measured amount of the drug and get it to the site of action quickly—especially if the route is intravenous. But injecting the drug is costly, unpleasant, and inconvenient. Many patients would not find the advantages worth it. Many would prefer a slower, less accurate delivery. They could choose among oral tablets, liquid, and perhaps other forms (such as nasal sprays, lozenges, suppositories, patches, and so forth). Each has advantages and disadvantages. Not everyone considering these options will hold values that lead to exactly the same choices.

Even if the physician can guess which dosage form is best for the patient, he or she still will have to determine the dose level, frequency of administration, and length of time the patient should take the drug. A patient with a severe arthritic attack might, if adequately informed, choose a short-term course of prednisone, a corticosteroid that is often effective in relieving the inflammation of the affected joint. The informed patient probably will want to taper the dose, because the prednisone affects the body's production of natural corticosteroids and stopping the drug cold turkey would produce a bodily backlash that almost anyone would find unacceptable. It would not be unreasonable, say, to go on a six-day course, taking, say, 30 mg the first day, 25 mg the second day, and so forth down to 5 mg on the last day. But if the patient wanted to increase the likelihood of overcoming the inflammation, he or she could start with a higher dose and taper more slowly, starting with, say, as much as 40 mg a day and tapering over a 10- or 12-day period down to 10 mg or less. Choosing the size of the dose and the number of days is not an exact science with only one possible answer. The more the patient fears the side effects of the prednisone, the smaller the dose and the shorter the regimen he or she will choose; the more he or she wants to attack the inflammation, the larger the dose and the longer the regimen. No easy way exists for the physician to know which choice is best for each individual patient.

Even if the physician can guess which approach is best for the patient, there still will be more choices to make. There may be more than one brand-name manufacturer, each with a different profile. One company may have a reputation for being very dependable, but expensive. Another may be cheaper, but a bit more suspect. There also may be generic manufacturers, some of which may be quite reliable, others unknown. Some patients may be morally committed to the generic market, believing that manufacturers that produce drugs at low cost and without advertising are providing a more useful service. Others may be militantly committed to the brand-name manufacturer, either because they believe they are more reliable or because they have a moral commitment to the idea that those companies put money into research and development and deserve to be rewarded for doing so.

Different physicians may make all of these choices somewhat differently. Because the choices are all independent of the pharmacological facts, it would be surprising if all physicians made these choices in exactly the same way. But there is no good reason why the patient should let these choices be made for her based on her physician's values and politics. Each of these choices should be made based on the patient's values, not those of the physician. Yet when a physician picks up a prescription pad and writes a prescription for a drug, it is the physician who typically makes all these choices. The physician often will actually write the "order" for the drug in such a way that it is illegible to the patient. "Sig: I tab tid po ac prn" means to the pharmacist, "Directions (sig), one (I) tablet (tab) three times a day (tid), by mouth (po), before meals (ac), as needed (prn)," but almost no patient understands this obscure Latin-based code.

Do physicians intentionally use this obscure code so that patients don't know what is being said? Sometimes they do, at least historically. The Hippocratic Oath actually required the physician to pledge that he would not reveal the secrets of medicine to the uninitiated layperson. The members of the Hippocratic cult believed that knowledge was potent and dangerous and that it should not fall into the hands of lay people.

John Wesley, the eighteenth-century founder of Methodism, was angry at physicians of his day for prescribing obscure and complex remedies.

He was even more hostile with pharmacists or apothecaries. As Wesley put it, "Experience shews, that one thing will cure most disorders, at least as well as twenty put together. Then why do you add the other nineteen? Only to swell the Apothecary's bill: nay, possibly, on purpose to prolong the distemper, that the Doctor and he may divide the spoil."[2]

When I was attending pharmacy school, I was taught that it was "unethical" for the pharmacist to explain the prescription to the patient because the physician might not want the patient to know what the doctor was doing.

That practice has fortunately changed to some degree. Now it is considered good practice to at least place the name of the drug on the prescription label. Patients are often told the name of the drug and its use, as well as reasonable side effects. Why, then, the continued use of the obscure code in writing prescriptions? Sometimes it is for speed and convenience. The string of abbreviations is shorthand that is quicker for the physician to write. It is also sometimes easier for the pharmacist to read. It may be easier to tell the difference in the physician's writing between "bid" and "tid" (twice-a-day and three-times-a-day, respectively) than the doctor's scrawled 2s and 3s. Sometimes, undoubtedly, the code still adds mystery and cachet to the practice of the physician. However, today there is no legitimate reason why the patient should not understand the exact content of the prescription and the instructions.

The real problem is more basic. The physician, faced with scores or even hundreds of variations in possible prescription elements (chemical, dose form, dosage, strength, manufacturer, and quantity), cannot possibly base all the choices on some mystical set of objective, scientific facts independent of the beliefs, values, and preferences of the patient. To write the prescription, the physician will need to explain the options to the patient and ask the patient which choice on each of the variables is best *for this patient*.

This means that the act of writing the prescription really should be the act of obtaining the patient's preferences and recording them. Prescribing should, at best, be the act of a *scribe*, of one who records the patient's choices. How, then, can we possibly justify laws that ban access to these thousands of drugs, unless the patient's scribe has written down the patient's choices?

Protecting Patients from Danger

A new era for medicine in which patients choose drugs available over-the-counter without prescription may, at first, sound too radical to be realistic.

After all, pharmaceuticals are more than just complex chemicals with potent effects, they are also potentially very dangerous, both to patients taking them for legitimate, orthodox medical reasons, and to others who may be the victims of abuse of drugs or of unorthodox, frivolous uses.

Of course, drugs are dangerous. They disrupt body chemistry in strange and unexplained ways. People can get hurt using them. In more traditional culture the only imaginable answer was to treat the patient as what people thought they were: uneducated, sometimes foolish decision makers, who, if left to their own choices, will likely hurt themselves. The proper answer was paternalism: constraining of people's autonomy for the purpose of protecting them from the harm they can do to themselves. The type of paternalism that was believed to be warranted was paternalism by physicians, physicians who would be given the authority by the state to control access to all manner of chemicals that were used as medicines (as well as other medical devices, therapies, and services such as surgery and radiation treatment).

In ancient culture this paternalism may have had some limited justification. Patients had, after all, much less education. They could not be expected to know what physicians knew. Moreover, because the cultures were more homogeneous, it would have been easier for the physician to guess the patient's values and therefore guess correctly what drugs the patient would have chosen had the patient been adequately knowledgeable. Most critically, ancient cultures generally were less troubled by paternalism. Greco-Roman culture did not have a well-developed doctrine of the individual and therefore was less concerned about what we might view as violations of individual rights. People did not protest violations of autonomy the way modern Americans might. Their circumstances led to paternalism in medicine and everything else in life.

Modern Western culture is radically different. In the United States, especially, the average layperson is much better educated, so he or she should be able to learn about and understand the treatment options, the risks and benefits, and other variables that need to be assessed based on the patient's value profile. This modern culture is also more diverse, more pluralistic. There is, therefore, much more room for physician error in guessing at the patient's value system. A tenth generation, WASP (white, Anglo-Saxon, Protestant) American male physician, who has a graduate-level education and is quite wealthy by world standards, might have a hard time imagining the value choices that would be made by a Black American teenage girl with a high-school education and different religious, cultural, social, and political commitments. Paternalism is a risky business in a pluralistic culture.

There still looms another problem with physician paternalism in pre-scription writing and other medical decision making. This kind of paternal-ism takes place without due process. Some lawyers with a soft spot in their hearts for paternalism indicate that some paternalism still exists even in American law. Jerry Menikoff, for example, points to present laws that pro-hibit access to drugs that have not been shown to be safe or effective.[3] He is merely pointing out, however, that American lawmakers can still be fooled into believing that choosing drugs is a task for medical experts who can make these choices based on science alone. Moreover, the laws to which he refers are surrounded with what lawyers call "legal due process." If a patient (or a manufacturer) believes that the FDA has been too restrictive in its la-beling decisions, there is a set of legal processes for public review. Judges can force overly paternalistic FDA officials to relax restrictions, and consum-ers have well-defined channels to challenge such paternalism. By contrast, paternalism by a physician in the privacy of the doctor's office is almost to-tally beyond due process.

Western liberal political philosophy is strongly committed to the princi-ple of autonomy of individuals in a way that ancient cultures were not. If paternalistic physicians are allowed to run roughshod over the free choices of a substantially autonomous person, those who subscribe to modern lib-eral individualism as a political philosophy will be offended in a way that their Greek and Roman—and even ancient Jewish and Christian—counter-parts were not. The risk of error is greater, and the offense is greater if an er-ror is made. When one combines these facts with the high likelihood that physicians will not know the proper values upon which to make prescribing choices, the dangers of medical paternalism become clear.

We should acknowledge that some members of postmodern society may still approve of paternalism, even paternalism by those who are not in a good position to know the patient's values. They may even approve of pa-ternalism without due process. Any competent patient has the right to turn over his or her decision-making responsibility to another person, and that person could be a physician. At least wise patients who know they are not well-informed about drug dangers would want the advice of a medical ex-pert on the possible benefits and harms of a drug. No one could complain if some people imposed on themselves a rule that they would not take medi-cations without being educated by a physician or even without the physi-cian's approval. The problem is that some people may not want to impose that restriction on themselves. They may be particularly worried about hav-ing to get the permission of someone who is more or less a stranger to them, who does not know their values, and who may hold values that are radically different from theirs. The real issue for the new era of medicine is whether adults who do not wish to be treated so paternalistically should be forced to endure such treatment. Once we realize that the physician who is writing the note that gives us permission to buy these drugs has no basis for knowing our values, such restrictions seem indefensible. As we shall see, even those who want to preserve the paternalism of traditional drug policies should insist on due process, and they should be willing to grant any patient access without the doctor's permission if the patient has a condition that will respond to the drug and has no special "contraindications" (special risks that would exclude use of the drug).

In no other area of twenty-first-century life do Americans stand to be treated in such a blatantly paternalistic way as in the act of physician drug prescribing practices. Even the physician who is, by now, committed to respecting patient autonomy—the one who would not imagine himself forcing treatment on Karen Quinlan if he knew it was against her will—will routinely pick up a prescription pad and write for a medication without any semblance of patient choice among treatment options.

Prescribing is an anachronism, a throwback to the paternalistic generation. Physicians have little, if any, basis for believing that once the full range of choices has been envisioned, they can really pick accurately what the patient would have chosen. They will often make plausible choices, at least based on their own values and perhaps based on the values held by the typical average citizen. But they are not prescribing for themselves or for typical, average citizens. They are prescribing for unique, individual patients. It is those patients who are in medical need and those patients who will pay the bill. The prescribing of medications and filling of prescriptions by pharmacists are acts that are no longer defensible. They should stop.

I say this as one who was trained in pharmacy and pharmacology. I say this as one who was a registered pharmacist for over 35 years (until I recently chose to "retire" from the career for which I was legally licensed but had not practiced for decades). This conclusion that prescribing makes no sense and should stop will undoubtedly offend many of my fellow pharmacists. It could jeopardize their livelihoods. It will undoubtedly offend many physicians as well, especially those who find psychological pleasure or remuneration from continuing in the paternalistic role. Being paid monthly to write renewal prescriptions for patients who need chronic medications has, for decades, been a lucrative business. Knowing that you are the "gatekeeper" for the nation's pharmaceuticals might be rewarding. But no matter how rewarding this role may, it is still indefensible. The practice of prescribing should stop.

THIRTEEN

The Alternatives to Prescribing

Two alternatives to requiring prescriptions from physicians to purchase any of thousands of pharmaceuticals are worth considering: the libertarian, free-market option and something I will call *patient certification*.

The Libertarian, Free-Market Alternative

One simple, bold alternative to the irrational practice of prescribing would be to bite the bullet and remove restrictions on medicinal chemicals: Let anyone sell them on the free market the way we sell nicotine, alcohol, pesticides, and countless other dangerous chemicals. As far as I know, there is no other class of products in the United States—a country passionately devoted to liberty—that is categorically restricted so that only a state-licensed professional (the pharmacist) may legally purchase and resell them, and only with written permission of another state-licensed professional (the physician). This is extraordinary security. It might be warranted for radioactive materials or top-secret, national-security data, but it is hard to defend for large classes of chemicals, most of which pose very little danger and have very little potential for abuse.

This, of course, is pharmaceutical heresy. The common wisdom is that drugs are complex, dangerous chemicals with which ordinary laypeople cannot be trusted. If people simply were permitted to walk into a store and buy them, we envision all manner of awful effects, both to the consumer and others. In fact, however, this vision of danger is too simple. Thousands of drugs restricted by federal food and drug law are relatively safe and pose, at most, a modest risk for abuse. They include hay fever medications, treatments for poison ivy, and angina drugs. Most pose essentially no temptation for abuse. If one does not have hay fever, poison ivy, or angina, these drugs are not very seductive. There are, of course, some exceptions, but the real fear of the traditional paternalist who advocates restriction usually is that people will intentionally hurt themselves or others if they are not supervised when these agents are used. Consider first the risks to other parties—the traditional domain of government restriction in a free society—before turning to the risk to the user.

Risks to Others

In a liberal society the one clear basis for coercive governmental restriction on the freedom of competent adults to lead their lives as they see fit is what is often referred to as the "harm" principle or, better, the "harm-to-others" principle. Even classical defenders of liberty, from the Founding Fathers to John Stuart Mill, recognized that if people are given the liberty to live their lives as they see fit, they may end up hurting others, either intentionally or accidentally. The state, in this classical liberal view, restricts the liberty of citizens when, and only when, the actions of the citizens will plausibly cause harm to others. Even then the standard interpretation holds that the harm to others must have a reasonable chance of occurring and that it will be more than trivial. One cannot falsely cry "fire" in a crowded theater, but one can build a fire on one's own property or even in a public space, provided the risk of the fire getting out of control and harming the interests of others is reasonably small.

In this classical liberal view, the state is within its rights to restrict drugs, chemicals, or any other agents that pose a significant danger to others. Many such dangerous agents come to mind: guns, knives, automobiles, and explosives, for example. Even many chemicals seem to fit: insecticide poisons, alcohol, and automobile antifreeze.

What is striking is how few classes of medicinal drugs fit. There are, of course, special cases: methamphetamine, narcotic analgesics, and antihistamines.

Methamphetamine and its chemical cousin, amphetamine, may be the clearest examples of medicinal drugs that pose some danger to others. When these chemicals are ingested, they may increase the likelihood of uncontrolled, violent behavior that threatens innocent third parties.

Narcotic analgesics (morphine, codeine, and many synthetic analogues) are often considered to pose an enormous risk—to both the user and others. The truth, as is often the case, is more complicated. There is no doubt that narcotic addicts must pay enormous sums to obtain a constant supply of their chemical on the illegal market, and they often have no means other than crime to obtain those resources. There is also no doubt that narcotic addiction corrupts the lives of people forced to lead this lifestyle, but that is primarily a risk not to others, but to the user himself or herself.

It is less clear that narcotic addiction poses any similar threat to the user or others when the drugs are obtained from a safe, cheap, legal source. A number of rather famous, socially responsible people have lived for periods of their lives as dependable, law-abiding citizens while addicted to narcotics. Sigmund Freud and one of the founders of the prestigious Johns Hopkins Medical School come to mind. Whether they were as creative, productive, and responsible as they would have been without the narcotic is debatable. No one has suggested, however, that they posed a serious danger to others.

Similarly, terminally and critically ill patients suffering from cancer and other painful, chronic conditions can be maintained indefinitely on narcotic analgesics without posing a danger to themselves or others, provided they have a reliable supply of their drug and do not rob, cheat, or steal to obtain it. The claim that narcotic analgesics must be restricted to protect people from themselves is a possibility that deserves long, serious reflection. The claim that they must be restricted to protect other parties is hard to sustain. Even if it can be sustained, it seems to pose a very limited harm-to-others exception to the libertarian's case for a free market in medicinal drugs.

There is one drug that clearly does pose a very serious threat to others: ethyl alcohol. Thousands of innocent people are killed every year from this single chemical. Hundreds of thousands of lives are seriously damaged by violent spousal abuse, inhibition-suppressed rape, assault, and lesser social offenses ranging from littering to indecent and offensive speech and public inconvenience. A very strong case still can be made for aggressive state restriction on markets in ethyl alcohol, notwithstanding the widespread belief that prohibition was a failure. In fact, the evidence that prohibition failed is harder to come by than most people realize. There is evidence that alcohol consumption decreased significantly and that many lives—including many innocent lives—were positively affected. Whether these benefits were really offset by the dangers from illegal behavior is hard to determine. Whether the need to protect others from the dangers of alcohol warranted constraint on the liberty of individual citizens is controversial to this day. One thing is clear: The legal efforts to prohibit purchase of alcohol were undertaken in the name of a philosophically justifiable moral principle—the harm-to-others principle. That is more than can be easily claimed for state controls on access to almost any other medicinal chemicals. Antihistamines, anti-inflammatory agents, and angina medications are not in the same league with alcohol. The risk to others, although capable of being imagined, is trivial in comparison.

Risk to the Patient

The truthful argument for the restriction on legend drugs (what we generally call "prescription" drugs) is not the well-defended harm-to-others principle; it is paternalistic. The goal is to protect people from themselves. That is in keeping with the ancient Hippocratic attitude, when individual rights and respect for the ordinary layperson were nearly nonexistent. That attitude is much harder to defend in the nation that prides itself on being the world's premier defender of liberty and justice for all. For those thousands of drugs that cannot possibly be feared as dangerous to innocent third parties, restriction on access by the Food and Drug Administration's cadre of experts is indefensible.

The doctrine of *caveat emptor* (let the buyer beware) is well known to twenty-first-century Americans. In fact, resting pharmaceuticals behind the protective barriers of the physician's prescription undoubtedly leaves consumers of medicinal drugs less attentive. They place their confidence in the judgment of a professional who they believe will protect them from danger and are therefore correspondingly less careful about making sure they know and understand the risks, drug interactions, and alternatives. This is so, even though the physician who is supposed to be protecting them may not have adequate knowledge of the patient's medical history, idiosyncratic reactions, and personal beliefs and values to know whether the prescribed drug poses an unacceptable risk of harm to the patient. Undoubtedly, if legend drugs were categorically removed from restriction, some laypeople would get hurt. But, just as certainly many consumers would quickly realize that they had a new responsibility to understand the risks and keep track of their own personal reactions.

If the decision were to be based solely on whether patients would face greater or less risk if drugs were sold on the free market without prescription, the consequences to the typical consumer of the drugs would be difficult to estimate. On the one hand, some patients undoubtedly would be injured.

On the other hand, laypeople would immediately have a strong incentive to take more responsibility for their medications. Some would even hire professional consultants or assistants to help them understand their medication choices. These professional assistants undoubtedly would be called "physicians." They might even be licensed by the state based on the state's assessment of their relevant expertise.

Although there are clear examples of persons being injured by inadequately educated medicinal choices, there are also clear cases of people being hurt because they cannot buy legend drugs on the open market.

CASE 13.1

The Vacationer Who Forgot His Medicine

A patient with a serious cardiac arrhythmia stabilized by the long-term use of the drug propranolol must take this medication every day. A precipitous interruption, once his body has adjusted to the medication, can cause a potentially fatal reaction. One such patient discovered, while traveling on vacation, that he had arrived in Florida one evening having left his propranolol at home. If he didn't take another dose by the next morning, he was at serious medical risk. He could not phone his pharmacy back home and have a new supply delivered to him. Even if he could reach his physician, that physician was not licensed to practice medicine in Florida and could not have legally transmitted a prescription for a refill. The patient's options were limited. He could go to a local emergency room, wait the standard, offensively long waiting time, and try to talk the stranger who finally cares for him into a new prescription for enough of the drug to get him through his vacation. The costs in time and money would have been substantial, not to mention the fact that the physician on duty in the emergency room is not in a good position to write the prescription in the first place. He simply would have to take the word of the patient about what medication and dose he was taking. The arrhythmia might not even be occurring at the time the patient was being seen by the physician. The physician would basically have to take the patient's word about the situation.

The patient also could go to a local pharmacist and try to talk the pharmacist into at least a few capsules to tide him over until he can get his supply from home. Providing even a few capsules on an emergency used to be illegal, but has now been legalized in some jurisdictions.

This option has only a limited chance of working and could place the pharmacist in some legal jeopardy.

Another option for the patient would be to ignore the problem and hope he does not suffer rebound arrhythmia in the morning. Considering the medical and financial costs and the inconvenience, this patient would have been much better off if he simply could have gone to the pharmacy and routinely bought a small bottle of the propranolol.

For each such story there is a counterexample of someone who might be hurt by permitting unlimited access, but libertarians claim that the interests and rights of these two groups of people do not have the same standing. They claim that in a liberal society, competent adults should be free to live their lives according to their own life plans and that this includes the right to buy and use anything, including drugs, that they can afford and for which they can find a willing seller, as long as the risks to third parties are controlled.

DRUGS FOR CHILDREN AND OTHER INCOMPETENT PERSONS

The most obvious rebuttal is to pose the problem of incompetent persons: children, mentally disabled adults, and others who lack the presumption of competency we usually attribute to normal adults. A free market in medicinal drugs without the doctor's written permission poses a problem for these people.

This is not a new problem in our society, however. There are many commodities that competent adults are allowed to purchase on the free market that they cannot legally transfer to children. Alcohol and tobacco are only the most obvious examples. Although adults can legally buy these products and use them, subject only to the constraints of the laws based in the harm-to-others principle, these adults cannot legally provide them to children.

Limits on Parental Freedom of Choice

Even though parents are required by the state to take responsibility for the welfare—including the health care—of their children, there are real constraints on how they may do so. Parents are permitted—indeed required—to make value judgments about how to promote their children's welfare, but they must act within reason. If they do not, the state will intervene. The parent will be accused of abuse or neglect—even if the abuse is undertaken in good faith.[1] Parents are not permitted to refuse life-saving blood transfusions or other medical treatments for their children, even if they are acting in good faith in doing so.[2] Christian Scientist parents cannot refuse to use a drug that will be life saving or substitute an alternative therapy that will seriously jeopardize their child's welfare. The state, even in a liberal society, has the clear power to prohibit parents from administering dangerous drugs to their children, even if those parents have the legal right to buy and use such drugs for themselves. There is no way that all the legend drugs in the world could do as much harm to children as parentally supplied alcohol has done, yet alcohol remains an over-the-counter drug freely available to adults.

A wise and tolerant state will exercise this control of parents cautiously. It permits parents to make a wide range of choices for the children, including some choices that are probably not the wisest. It permits parents to choose a school system, for instance. Parents can choose public school, parochial school, military school, private nonsectarian school, or avant garde experimental school, even though, in some cases, some of these options clearly are not the best for their children. The state would be too burdened if it had to monitor every such choice. As one court said, "It is fundamental that parental autonomy is constitutionally protected. The United States Supreme Court has articulated the concept of personal liberty found in the Fourteenth Amendment as a right of privacy which extends to certain aspects of a family relationship."[3]

A similar position was adopted by The President's Commission for the Study of Ethical Problems in Medicine and Biomedical and Behavioral Research in its report on *Deciding to Forego Life-Saving Treatment:* "This society has traditionally been very reluctant to intrude upon the functioning of families, both because doing so would be difficult and because it would also destroy some of the value of the family which seems to need a fair degree of privacy and discretion to maintain its significance."

Applied to the parental decision maker, parents are given wide-ranging discretion in the decisions they make for their children. They are permitted to make choices that some people would consider inappropriate as long as the deviation from the most plausible decisions does not amount to abuse or neglect.

The state has ample authority to intervene when it has to. It could and would limit the right of parents to give their children dangerous medicinal drugs.

That Pediatricians Are Not Parents

Given that the state would have to place limits on parental authority for children's drug use, why not, some might ask, just give that authority back to the pediatrician so that the child's doctor would become the agent for the state to determine when drugs should be used? It could do so if it chose, but this seems unwise. The choice of drugs is, as we have seen, a value choice. It is the parents, not the pediatrician, who have the authority to exercise discretion in making these value choices for their children. It is the parents' values, not the pediatrician's, that should be imposed on the child. The state would have the option of reeducating pediatricians to oversee parental use of dangerous drugs for the children. But it would require teaching pediatricians the subtleties of their new role. They would no longer be charged with determining when the use of a certain drug was in the child's best interest. Rather, they would be charged with reviewing the parental choice and estimating whether the parents have gone beyond reason in deciding which drugs their child should be using. Even then, it is not clear why a pediatrician, a private citizen with no moral authority over the child, should be designated by the state to exercise its *parens patriae* authority. The task is to make, on behalf of the state, the value judgment about when parents have deviated too severely from what the state considers the child's best interest. There is no reason why the pediatrician should be good at making that value judgment or why this health professional should know how much discretion is too much. That is why we rely on the courts, not physicians, to be the ultimate authority in overruling parental drug choices. At least the courts operate with due process, checks over deviant judgments, and a rule of law that limits judges' authority.

Thus, a bold, simple free market in legend drugs is harder to oppose than it might seem. Clear medical and economic advantages would result, even if there would be offsetting disadvantages. The real issue is whether our society is sufficiently committed to the principles of liberty to give competent adults the freedom to make these choices for themselves when the harm-to-others principle does not come into play. Because children and other incompetents would be protected, it is hard to see what moral ground there is for this dramatic constraint on human freedom in a matter that is literally life-and-death. Nevertheless, some will doubt that the United States is sufficiently committed to human freedom to attempt this radical experiment. For them, and I may be included in this group, there is a second alternative.

Patient Certification as an Alternative to Prescribing

If we are too timid to move all drugs currently restricted to prescription use to an over-the-counter free market, there is a more cautious option. We could permit adults to buy legend drugs from pharmacies only after the patient has been certified to be an adequate consumer. This way, we could ensure that everyone who purchased these supposedly dangerous chemicals knew enough about the risks, benefits, precautions, and alternatives to protect themselves against the dangers. Certification could come in several forms. The main options include certification for competence and certification for diagnosis.

Either or both could be used effectively. Either would be a significant improvement, not only in assuring human freedom in an area fundamentally important to life, but also in making the drug user a competent, responsible consumer. It would be a vast improvement over the traditional passive role of the patient, who blindly took whatever medications the doctor ordered. It would even be an improvement over the current model in which the patient is supposed to be informed about the uses and risks of the drug and is supposed to consent to them. Presently, there is no requirement that the patient be certified as competent to use the medication he or she is given. That judgment continues to rest primarily with the physician. If patients had to have a certificate testifying to the appropriateness of their skills and diagnosis, then they ought to be better, more active consumers.

CERTIFYING COMPETENCE

Certifying competence is the more important and less controversial option. If defenders of traditional prescription writing are concerned that a free market in legend drugs would lead to uninformed purchases, the most straightforward response is to require that the patient be tested and certified for this competence. The one doing the certifying might even be the same physician who under the current system has the authority to prescribe—to choose a drug and authorize its use. The form on which the certificate was written undoubtedly would look very much like the present prescription, but its nature would be very different. The piece of paper signed by the physician would not prescribe; it would certify that the patient has been found adequately competent to decide whether to buy and use a certain medication. It would be a public testimony of the physician's opinion of the patient's competence with regard to the medication and its use. It is no longer a permission; it is a testament.

Some might worry that the patient certified to be competent might still exercise poor judgment and refuse to take medication that would be beneficial. That is, of course, a risk, but it is a risk that already exists in our current policy. Doctors presently complain about patients who do not fill prescriptions.

In fact, no patient is required to take the medication prescribed by the physician. We presently live in the crazy half-libertarian world in which patients are not considered capable of deciding on their own to take medications, but are considered capable of refusing to take medications prescribed by their physicians. Refusing to take medications can be at least as dangerous as taking the wrong drugs. People die daily because they refuse medications—sometimes intentionally, sometimes without understanding what they are doing. We generally believe that this is the price we pay for living in a free society. As long as a person is mentally competent and the drug is prescribed for the patient's own good, his or her right to refuse is unlimited. In fact, there has never been a case in American law (at least not any that have not been overturned on appeal) in which a competent American has ever been forced to take a drug offered for the patient's own good. Why the liberty to consume doesn't match the liberty to refuse is a mystery.

CERTIFYING DIAGNOSIS

Some still would fear that this could result in some patients buying and using medications for "unauthorized" purposes. Because medications can be dangerous or useless for people with one condition, even if they are exactly right for someone with another, merely certifying competence might not completely do the job of protecting the patient from misuse of the drug. Those with lingering paternalistic inclinations may want the world structured so that the patient, even the adequately informed and certified patient, cannot get access to a drug when that drug is not seen as appropriate for the patient's condition.

The easy solution would be to add a second type of certification—certification for diagnosis. This would require a physician to certify that the patient has been diagnosed with a condition for which the drug is appropriate. This way, a patient would not be able to go to the store and buy an antibiotic for a viral infection, because antibiotics are not effective for treating them. Only if the patient could be diagnosed with a bacterial infection known to be amenable to the antibiotic would a certificate be issued.

This would be a policy far superior to the current arrangement. There is no rule, law, or policy requiring physicians to prescribe drugs only for conditions for which the drug has been shown to be effective. The physician confronting a patient who demands a prescription for an antibiotic for what the physician has good reason to believe to be a viral infection, can today prescribe the antibiotic. Under present norms good physicians would not do so, but some do. They do so to get rid of a patient who is a nuisance or to generate additional income from the charge for writing the prescription. A policy requiring certification for diagnosis would eliminate this abuse.

A certificate for diagnosis would pose an interesting problem. It would require a master list of which drugs can be used for which diagnoses. Producing such a list would be a monumental and controversial task, but it is implied in the belief that patients can use drugs only for diagnoses that conform to some external standard. It would be fun watching medical experts trying to come up with such a list.

Critics actually may object to the proposal to certify by diagnosis, precisely because they believe it is important to retain a certain amount of freedom to try drugs for diagnoses beyond those for which there is widespread agreement that the drug is appropriate. They value the physician's freedom to exercise "clinical judgment" in special cases. It was once widely believed that no objective list of treatments, even one based on a complex diagnostic and treatment protocol, could match the individual clinician's subtle, individualized judgment for the patient. Even two decades ago, however, scholars began to realize that carefully crafted treatment protocols added greatly to the clinician's individual judgment. In 1980, a collection of essays had already been published that put forward the claim that a protocol—that is, a standard set of decision-making rules—could outperform the typical clinician.[4] That was before the era of computers. By now, with new, formal treatment protocols, if we are to limit access to drugs by diagnosis, a formally developed list with adequate public review and time for revision will certainly be superior to the gut-feeling, intuitive judgment of the individual practitioner.

There is another kind of problem. Many people believe that in addition to the standard uses for medications, clinicians should have the freedom to prescribe for "unapproved uses" for patients who have unusual conditions or have not responded to standard therapies. The concept of an "unapproved use" is a slippery one, however. The FDA does not actually approve "uses" for drugs, and therefore there is no universal standard for what the approved uses are. What the FDA does is approve labeling. A manufacturer cannot claim on its label that the drug is used ("indicated") for a condition unless it has adequate scientific evidence to support the claim. If a chemical has not received FDA approval for any use, it is illegal to transport the drug in interstate commerce. Unless one is willing to work entirely within one state (an implausible limitation for drug manufacturers today), the agent cannot be marketed, and therefore no physician can use it.

However, once a drug has had labeling approved for some one use, it can be shipped in interstate commerce and pharmacists can stock it. Physicians may legally prescribe it, *even for a use that is not on the label*. Some unlabeled uses are for medical problems in which the drug is widely known or at least believed to be effective, but for scientific or economic reasons the manufacturer has simply never bothered to develop and submit the data to the FDA to back up that belief. Physicians may, with relative lack of controversy, prescribe for these "unlabeled conditions."

More controversial is the practice of novel "off-label" uses by physicians. Any physician who has a hunch that a drug may be beneficial for a condition for which it has never been tried may legally prescribe that drug, as long as the drug is on the market for some other use. There is no requirement for the physician to get permission or approval. The naive patient may receive the prescription not knowing it to be a wild idea in the imagination of his or her physician. The physician is merely subject to the normal rules of malpractice, which hold that if a patient is injured, the physician may be financially liable. Most novel uses that have their origin in the minds of innovative practitioners never hurt anybody, and so no lawsuit is filed. Even if the patient is directly injured by the novel use, he or she may have no idea what caused the problem and therefore would not complain. It is a crazy policy designed to avoid offending physicians who are a powerful political group who get annoyed if a government agency tells them how to practice medicine, but no legal limits are placed on physicians who prescribe for off-label uses, even implausible and indefensible ones. For some bizarre reason the deviant physician is permitted to draw on his or her oddball values in prescribing a treatment for a patient, but the patient is not given the same freedom to purchase drugs based on his or her own values—even when the patient can be certified as suffering from a condition for which the drug is known to be useful.

Now the question arises whether requiring a certificate for diagnosis would undercut this practice of off-label physician prescribing. The answer depends on how the list of approved diagnoses is constructed. If the list of diagnoses exactly matched the FDA's list of labeled uses, then all the off-label uses would be excluded. One could envision a list based on a looser standard that included recognized off-label uses, even though the FDA had not been convinced to include the uses in its labeling. The real underlying question is what our national policy ought to be regarding off-label uses.

The present policy permits physicians to prescribe for off-label uses (subject only to normal medical malpractice constraints if the physician injures the patient by prescribing for such use). The physician is legally free to prescribe any currently available drug for any possible use. The FDA even goes so far as to defend the physician's right to do so, claiming it is not within the scope of its authority to practice medicine. By doing so the FDA decreases the wrath of the physician community, avoiding offending a critically powerful constituency.

The present policy seems completely irrational and indefensible. If an agent is on the market for some labeled use for which the FDA has received adequate data to deem it safe and effective for that use, then the individual physician can use that same drug for some other diagnosis, even though there have never been any studies showing it is effective or even safe. Some drugs that are clearly safe and effective for some medical conditions can be useless or even dangerous for some other condition. There is no a priori reason to believe that the drug will be safe or effective for any condition just because it has been shown to be so for one well-studied problem. The same paternalistic logic that leads to the law banning drugs from interstate commerce until they have been shown to be safe and effective for one use should, from the paternalistic point of view, require banning their use for other conditions for which there is not adequate evidence of safety and efficacy.

On the other hand, if the paternalism of the old prescribing rituals is indefensible and we should shift to a buyer-beware market, the same policy would seem right for drugs that have not yet been found either safe or effective for their first use. Either we should ban use of a drug until it is found safe and effective for any given use or we should permit access without safety and efficacy data for that use. We cannot logically have it both ways.

If we accept the idea that people should be able to obtain drugs for off-label uses (at least when standard treatments have proven ineffective and patients are adequately informed), then it should not matter whether the drug happens to be labeled for some other use. If we are to permit off-label uses, however, it is hard to imagine why the discretion should rest on the whim of the physician. Perhaps paternalists should support a formal government agency with review powers and authority to come up with a standard list of uses that are plausible, even though adequate data are not available to support labeling. Perhaps libertarians should support giving such discretion to individual patients who, after being adequately informed of the reasons for trying the drug, would be allowed to choose to use the drug for a diagnosis not on the label. What seems totally implausible is giving this discretion to individual physicians.

Paternalists should accept the idea that a drug should be available for a particular diagnosis when enough data exist for the FDA to add it to its list of diagnoses. Antipaternalists should believe in freedom enough to allow their fellow citizens to make these decisions for their own cases. But how can anyone let the patient be exposed to an off-label use if his or her private physician has beliefs and values supporting the use while we know that another physician facing the same patient with exactly the same facts would make a choice against the off-label use? The frustrated patient who wants the drug is forced to doctor shop until he or she finds the doctor with the right gut feelings, beliefs, values, and moral commitments. Eventually, the patient might find a doctor willing to do what the patient has chosen, but that surely makes no sense. It is far better to give the patient the decision-making authority, at least within a range of plausible uses.

Certifying by diagnosis would, in effect, reproduce a set of behaviors that are familiar. The patient would visit a physician. The physician would diagnose and review certain treatment options. Instead of prescribing the one that the physician thinks best, subject only to the patient's informed consent, the physician would certify the patient's competence to purchase the drug and perhaps certify that the patient has a diagnosis for which the drug is suitable. The certificate would look very much like a prescription, but it would be very different conceptually. It would be a testimony of condition and competence, not an order (or even a recommendation) for a treatment. The patient would then review his or her options and decide whether to visit a store and buy the medication. The pharmacist would counsel, review the physician's actions, and dispense (or sell) the medication, much as he or she does now. The result, however, would be a very new set of transactions and authority patterns. The patient would choose whether to use a drug instead of doing what the doctor says. If the libertarian free market is too radical an idea, certified buyers of drugs may be an interim alternative.

A SPECIAL EXCEPTION FOR ABUSABLE DRUGS?

This option still leaves open the problem of the small group of drugs that are really dangerous: the ones that can cause real harms to third parties. It might also include the ones that pose serious risk of abuse for the user himself or herself. We have seen that this is a very small group of exceptions indeed: amphetamines, narcotics, and alcohol being the most plausible cases of drugs dangerous to others, and a handful of drugs that are really dangerous to the patient who takes them. There can be no real objection to the policy of imposing strict, nonpaternalistic controls on access to drugs that are really dangerous to others. Whether that includes narcotics or only amphetamines and alcohol is a question that will have to be left to public debate. Those that are really dangerous to others certainly should be controlled. I would favor such controls on amphetamines, alcohol, and perhaps narcotics as well.

It is also possible that some drugs are unusually risky for the user or are subject to uses that the society finds unacceptable. The same propranolol that we discussed as a treatment for patients with serious cardiac arrhythmia can, for example, be taken by public speakers and actors to treat stage fright. A policy permitting open-market access without certification of diagnosis would make the drug available not only to people with heart problems, but also those who are afraid to go on stage. If the society were really offended by this use, as they might be offended by the use of RU-486 to produce abortion, for example, then it might temporarily abandon its constitutional dedication to liberty and retreat to paternalism to ban access to them. Suspending constitutional liberties to prevent someone from preventing stage fright or even to prevent an abortion is a momentous choice. I hope it would not happen.

| Are Fat People Overweight?

A few years ago, the National Institutes of Health (NIH)—the federal government's medical research institute complex in Bethesda, Maryland, and the most famous medical research facility in the world—issued a set of weight "standards" that labeled anyone with a body mass index greater than 25 as "overweight" and anyone with an index greater than 30 as "obese."[1] The BMI takes into account both weight and height: Body weight in kilograms is divided by the square of one's height expressed in meters. The authors believe the goal is to have a BMI below 25. Thus, by these federal guidelines, anyone 5′9″ tall should weigh less than 169 lbs. and anyone 5′4″ tall 145 lbs. regardless of gender. One study that group relied on concludes that in the United States 54.9 percent of adults are overweight or obese.

Any bureaucracy that can count overweight and obese people so precisely must have some very specific criteria in mind. It should arouse one's curiosity. They talk as if being overweight or obese were an objective medical condition that a physician can diagnose and treat based on medical science. Medical publications and credible lay press tout the harms from being overweight. Even the ones that are carefully edited use *fat* and *overweight* interchangeably. But they have no idea how to tell the difference between being "fat" and being "overweight."

Body Mass Index Table

	Normal						Overweight					Obese										Extreme Obesity														
BMI	19	20	21	22	23	24	25	26	27	28	29	30	31	32	33	34	35	36	37	38	39	40	41	42	43	44	45	46	47	48	49	50	51	52	53	54
Height (inches)												Body Weight (pounds)																								
58	91	96	100	105	110	115	119	124	129	134	138	143	148	153	158	162	167	172	177	181	186	191	196	201	205	210	215	220	224	229	234	239	244	248	253	258
59	94	99	104	109	114	119	124	128	133	138	143	148	153	158	163	168	173	178	183	188	193	198	203	208	212	217	222	227	232	237	242	247	252	257	262	267
60	97	102	107	112	118	123	128	133	138	143	148	153	158	163	168	174	179	184	189	194	199	204	209	215	220	225	230	235	240	245	250	255	261	266	271	276
61	100	106	111	116	122	127	132	137	143	148	153	158	164	169	174	180	185	190	195	201	206	211	217	222	227	232	238	243	248	254	259	264	269	275	280	285
62	104	109	115	120	126	131	136	142	147	153	158	164	169	175	180	186	191	196	202	207	213	218	224	229	235	240	246	251	256	262	267	273	278	284	289	295
63	107	113	118	124	130	135	141	146	152	158	163	169	175	180	186	191	197	203	208	214	220	225	231	237	242	248	254	259	265	270	278	282	287	293	299	304
64	110	116	122	128	134	140	145	151	157	163	169	174	180	186	192	197	204	209	215	221	227	232	238	244	250	256	262	267	273	279	285	291	296	302	308	314
65	114	120	126	132	138	144	150	156	162	168	174	180	186	192	198	204	210	216	222	228	234	240	246	252	258	264	270	276	282	288	294	300	306	312	318	324
66	118	124	130	136	142	148	155	161	167	173	179	186	192	198	204	210	216	223	229	235	241	247	253	260	266	272	278	284	291	297	303	309	315	322	328	334
67	121	127	134	140	146	153	159	166	172	178	185	191	198	204	211	217	223	230	236	242	249	255	261	268	274	280	287	293	299	306	312	319	325	331	338	344
68	125	131	138	144	151	158	164	171	177	184	190	197	203	210	216	223	230	236	243	249	256	262	269	276	282	289	295	302	308	315	322	328	335	341	348	354
69	128	135	142	149	155	162	169	176	182	189	196	203	209	216	223	230	236	243	250	257	263	270	277	284	291	297	304	311	318	324	331	338	345	351	358	365
70	132	139	146	153	160	167	174	181	188	195	202	209	216	222	229	236	243	250	257	264	271	278	285	292	299	306	313	320	327	334	341	348	355	362	369	376
71	136	143	150	157	165	172	179	186	193	200	208	215	222	229	236	243	250	257	265	272	279	286	293	301	308	315	322	329	338	343	351	358	365	372	379	386
72	140	147	154	162	169	177	184	191	199	206	213	221	228	235	242	250	258	265	272	279	287	294	302	309	316	324	331	338	346	353	361	368	375	383	390	397
73	144	151	159	166	174	182	189	197	204	212	219	227	235	242	250	257	265	272	280	288	295	302	310	318	325	333	340	348	355	363	371	378	386	393	401	408
74	148	155	163	171	179	186	194	202	210	218	225	233	241	249	256	264	272	280	287	295	303	311	319	326	334	342	350	358	365	373	381	389	396	404	412	420
75	152	160	168	176	184	192	200	208	216	224	232	240	248	256	264	272	279	287	295	303	311	319	327	335	343	351	359	367	375	383	391	399	407	415	423	431
76	156	164	172	180	189	197	205	213	221	230	238	246	254	263	271	279	287	295	304	312	320	328	336	344	353	361	369	377	385	394	402	410	418	426	435	443

Source: Adapted from Clinical Guidelines on the Identification, Evaluation, and Treatment of Overweight and Obesity in Adults: The Evidence Report

FIGURE 14.1 Body Mass Index. (Reprinted from National Institutes of Health, National Heart, Lung, and Blood Institute, *Clinical Guidelines on the Identification, Evaluation, and Treatment of Overweight and Obesity in Adults: The Evidence Report*. NIH Publication No. 98-4083. http://www.nhlbi.nih.gov/guidelines/obesity/bmi_tbl.pdf.)

Fat versus Overweight

Fat, as it is usually applied to humans, is a descriptive term characterizing people who are significantly above the average weight for their height. I know. We still have to make a judgment about how far one is above the average before he or she becomes fat. I know. Fat has to be defined with regard to some reference group. The fattest person in the Nazi concentration camps was still thin; the thinnest Sumo wrestler is still fat. But to say someone is fat should convey nothing more than a fact—a fact about a person's weight taking into account his or her height. No value judgment need be implied. It is linguistically possible to say of someone that the person is "fat," without claiming that that person is too heavy. Although it is not common usage, he or she can be said to be fat and the "right weight" simultaneously without linguistic contradiction. In the new medicine that this book is about, a person can be fat and at his ideal weight at the same time. This chapter explains why.

Saying someone is *overweight*, however, is different. Saying someone is overweight is a value judgment. A person can't be overweight and be the right weight at the same time. It is striking that the NIH report defines "overweight" two ways. One is simply quantitative: A person is overweight—by definition—whenever the BMI is above 25. This first definition seems clearly to be incorrect usage. It would be remarkable if in all the world everyone became overweight at exactly the same body mass index. Crossing the BMI 25 threshold might trigger the descriptor "fat" or "obese" or "plump," but it seems odd to apply these terms in such a rigid numerical manner. Most importantly, it is theoretically possible that someone with a BMI over 25 was exactly at his or her ideal weight.

The second definition is that a person has *excess* weight.[2] Embedded in the term is a standard—an ideal or "right" weight that the person has exceeded. That clearly is a value judgment, not a fact. One cannot have "excess weight" and be at one's ideal weight at the same time.

Scientists are taught that they are not supposed to make these kinds of value judgments when they are reporting facts. To claim someone has excess weight is to claim that there is some negative value attached to these weights, something to worry about. The problem is that it is not the role of science to tell us what we should worry about in life. That is the role of cultures, religions, or—even better—individuals.

Reasons to Worry about Weight

There are really only three reasons to worry about being overweight. The first two are legitimate; the third is the one on everyone's mind. First, most people believe that heavier people (people who are heavy for their height) are at risk of dying prematurely. Second, most people also believe that being fat makes people feel worse than they would if they were thinner. They believe we have more disease risk, joint problems, shortness of breath, and generally just feel worse. We will look at the link between weight and these medical risks in the following chapter. First, however, let's look at the social rewards of being thin.

What's on most people's minds has nothing to do with dying or the physical discomforts of carrying the weight. It's a fear that others won't think they look pretty. (For males, we usually use other words, such as handsome or good-looking, but, for our purposes, they all refer to socially imposed standards that convey approval of one's physical appearance.) Those who aren't pretty are supposed to fear that they won't impress friends, family, and work colleagues with their attractiveness. They may even fear they won't make as much money, be offered as good a job, or find as desirable a mate.[3] Before we take on the supposed risk of death and disease from being fat, we need to confront the *prettiness argument* head on.

The Value of Being Pretty

Most people who are honest about why they are trying to lose weight will admit that they are not primarily trying to protect their health. They are trying to conform to some social or cultural ideal about what is pretty. They are seeking the social rewards for being thin, which, in our culture, are enormous. The skinny get the most appealing dates, marital partners, friends, and even jobs. For some people these rewards are so attractive that they are worth almost any torture that perpetual dieting can cause.

Some adolescents (particularly adolescent girls) place such value on thinness that they will do almost anything—take any risk—to pursue it. For them anorexia is not a disease, nor is bulimia. These are treatments for the disease of not being pretty. They are treatments for diseases of the immature and socially insecure (even if the person is named Diana and happens to know that she could become the future queen of England). Looking pretty for others is simply not a standard that the NIH has any business propagating.

I don't fault insecure adolescents who want to look pretty for others. No doubt for some people, much satisfaction accrues from pursuing the rewards of pop culture. But for some of us, there is more to life than these pursuits. We are adequately secure, adequately mature (or adequately ugly) that the rewards of the quest for social approval of our prettiness are not satisfying. We have adequate self-confidence. Or at least we don't care enough to pursue the "ideal" of being skinny.

Now, of course, not all people below the BMI of 25 are skinny. In fact, the NIH report indicates that one must drop below a BMI of 18.5 before one becomes too thin. That would be under about 110 pounds for someone 5'4" tall. These people are labeled "underweight." They face the same problem as the "overweight." They have to conform to the socially imposed standard or risk being ostracized.

Within these boundaries between a body mass index of 18.5 and 25 are the people who the society and NIH would have us believe are "just right." The question is how do they know what is just right? Why is prettiness below 25 pretty enough, but prettiness below 18.5 "sick"? Why should those of us who are fat consider ourselves overweight? In the next chapter, we will look at the other reasons to be concerned about weight: the risk of death and disease.

| Beyond Prettiness

Death, Disease, and Being Fat

The guidelines for so-called ideal weight were prepared by the National Institutes of Health. They don't claim to be concerned about prettiness. They
need to have health-related reasons for considering fat people overweight
and superskinny people sick. They believe that being overweight is bad for
your health and that when something is bad for your health it is bad for
you. Hence, the other two reasons people might be concerned about weight—
mortality and morbidity, that is, death and poor health.

Oddly, the NIH report never actually shows that anything bad happens
when one crosses the line to the BMI of 25. Believe it or not, the entire report does not ever show that things begin to get worse at this point. One
might guess that the people at the NIH think either that a BMI of 25 is the
point at which things begin to happen that they consider to be bad or that
this is the point at which the rate of increase in bad health effects gets to be
so great that they believe it is time to take weight seriously. The report
clearly shows that higher BMIs are related to some medical consequences
that most people think are bad. It does not, however, show that these consequences start right at a BMI of 25 or that these consequences are bad. It
does not even show that the larger body mass causes these problems.

The Supposed Risk of Death

Most people, including most medical experts, believe that being fat speeds death. They make what seems like a reasonable assumption that it is not good to die, and they conclude that it is better to be thin. But that reasoning is too fast. Does being heavy really increase the death risk, and does lowering body weight actually lower that risk? Most critically, is living as long as possible really the ultimate goal of living?

DOES BEING HEAVY INCREASE
THE DEATH RISK?

Heavier people do appear to have an increased mortality risk. Reliable studies have shown increased risk of adenocarcinoma of the esophagus,[1] pancreatic cancer,[2] and, many other forms of cancer.[3] Similar findings show higher risk of stroke at high BMI.[4] A study published a few years ago in the *Journal of the American Medical Association* concludes that 280,000 deaths a year are attributable to what it calls overweight and obesity among U.S. adults.[5] The authors examine six major, respected studies upon the basis of which they can estimate the number of deaths they attribute to weight. The situation is actually worse. Some overweight people are also smokers, and they die of smoking before their obesity can get them. The authors estimate that 325,000 deaths would be attributable to obesity if it were not for the smoking. The well-known and respected National Health and Nutrition Examination Survey (NHANES) estimated 111,909 excess deaths from obesity (BMI greater than 30) in the year 2000.[6]

We need not be so defensive about this that we deny that weight is associated with increased mortality, but these conclusions still need to be examined. Some studies in distinguished medical journals present a more complicated picture. One *New England Journal of Medicine* study, for example, found, for white subjects, small increases in the risk of death as body mass index increased and that the risks, as expected, got greater as BMI got to be very high. For African-American subjects, however, death risk actually was lower for people in the BMI range of 25 to 28 than it was for those in the 23.5–24.9 range. Moreover, even though death risk increased at higher BMI ranges, even in the highest group, the difference was not statistically significant.[7] Another study showed years of life lost at higher BMI numbers, but similarly found no detrimental effect in blacks until BMI reached the low thirties for men and high thirties for women. Moreover, even though there were detrimental effects at the highest BMI ranges, the time lost from obesity was small for older persons, measured in months or, at most, a year or two, and for older Blacks higher BMI actually correlated with a gain in years of life.[8] The NHANES study did not find excess mortality for those they classified as "overweight" (i.e., a BMI between 25 and 30). Actually, they found less mortality, but the difference was not statistically significant. For those who had never smoked, the risk was less for overweight than so-called ideal weight persons in the age group 25–29, and if there was an increased death risk, it never reached statistical significance for most age groups.[9]

The authors of the NIH report come very close to making an unforgivable error for a scientist: claiming that when two events are associated, we know that one of them causes the other. The authors say that the excess deaths are "attributed" to obesity. They may be right. In fact, it is a good guess. But their data do not prove that the obesity causes these deaths. A correlation—an association—is not a cause. Sometimes two associated factors may themselves result from some unmeasured third factor that causes both. Deaths from drowning seem to go up at the same time as the sale of ice cream, but ice cream is probably not the cause of the drowning (nor does the drowning cause ice cream sales). Some third factor—the weather—undoubtedly causes both.

It seems plausible that when studies consistently show that fatter people die sooner, their fat is causing the deaths. But so far that's just a guess. Many other explanations are possible. For example, a study of the relation of BMI and cardiovascular disease in women found people with higher BMI numbers had more cardiovascular disease, but these people also tended to be less physically fit. When fitness was taken into account, the relation between BMI and cardiovascular disease disappeared.[10]

Genes affect virtually all bodily functions. Genes tend to make us have heart disease and cancer. Genes also control our body frames and our weight.[11] It is possible that the genes that are responsible for lethal diseases are associated with those that control our body frames.[12] If these genes are near each other on a chromosome, people who inherit the gene for heart disease or cancer also could inherit the gene for being fat.

If this is true, reducing weight would not by itself eliminate the genes for the death-inducing diseases. Making people as skinny as Karen Carpenter would just allow them to be skinny when they die prematurely from heart attacks.

Or consider another hypothesis: It could be that fat people have certain personality traits that also lead them to behaviors that make them die sooner—regardless of their weight. Among these traits might be a love of motorcycle riding or beer drinking, for instance. Someone with a personality that generates a slovenly, happy-go-lucky attitude indifferent to social opinion may have a trait that both makes them fat and increases their risk for death. Fixing the fatness would still leave a skinny guy who takes risky motorcycle rides and chugs beer. What we need to know is whether getting fat people to reduce their weight will, by itself, cause them to live longer.

In a little noticed section of the NIH report, the authors actually admit something surprising. They state, "In most, but not all, of these studies, generic weight loss and weight cycling are associated with increases in mortality."[13] That's right, weight loss is associated with *increase* in mortality. This doesn't mean very much because some weight loss may be unintentional, even related to the existence of serious diseases, but at least they are not claiming that there is evidence that weight loss reduces mortality.

The report cites three studies that focus on the relation of *intentional* weight loss and mortality. The first might appear to provide evidence that weight loss actually reduces mortality, the result the naive person might expect. It was conducted in India on patients who had had heart attacks and whose weight was, on average, normal. Those who lost at least one pound had a 54 percent lower overall mortality after one year compared to those who did not.[14] The result is ambiguous because these people were not selected because they were heavy to begin with. It is also puzzling that such a small change in weight could be responsible for such a dramatic difference in mortality. It is hard to know what to make of such dramatic findings from people who were not obese to begin with, especially when one adds the other two studies.

The second study involved 43,000 American women aged 60–64 who had never smoked. Among those with obesity-related medical problems (diabetes and other conditions known to be made worse by weight), those who intentionally lost any amount of weight not surprisingly had a 20 percent reduction in overall mortality, but among those without these medical problems, a loss of 20 pounds in a year's time was associated with "small to modest *increases* in mortality."[15]

The third study included obese men and women in Sweden, some of whom had self-selected for surgery for purposes of weight reduction. The NIH analysts project that the group that chose surgery will eventually have 10-year mortality that is lower, perhaps because of greater weight loss.[16] This is in part due to reduction in diabetes and lipid levels. The problem here, however, is that a group that chooses voluntarily to have surgery to deal with their health problems are almost certainly more motivated than those who do not. It is very hard to tell whether the projected improvement in mortality is caused by the greater weight reduction or by some other behavior changes that these people have chosen. They might, for instance, have lowered their lipids and controlled their diabetes better regardless of weight loss. They might have been more inclined to exercise.

Mortality may only be associated with increased weight and not caused by it. If so, getting fat people thinner will do nothing to lower their mortality risk. If that is the case, the authors of the NIH and the *JAMA* studies (and virtually all physician advice about weight loss) are mistaken.

WILL LOWERING WEIGHT EXTEND LIFE?

If fat people lower their weight, will they live longer? I have seen dozens of studies showing that fat people die sooner, but in spite of having searched for years, the evidence just mentioned is the best I have ever seen to try to show that lowering fat people's weight makes them live longer. A proper study would be one conducted on very large samples, probably thousands of people, divided randomly into two groups. The members of one group would be assigned the task of lowering their weight, whereas the members of the other group would function as a control. If, after many years, the first group had lowered their weight more than the control group and also had a lower mortality, that would be evidence that being fat caused the excess mortality. An uncontrolled study will not do. If a group lowers its weight and its mortality declines without having a control group, something else may have caused the drop in deaths. For example, pollution or infectious disease may have been reduced or physicians may have gotten better at preventing deaths from heart disease.

A study in Finland comes as close as anything I know to being a controlled study. The control group was not random, so the results are controversial, but the outcome is provocative. The study involved twins. It followed 2,957 people with a body mass equal to or higher than 25, the NIH fat police standard for being overweight. In 1975 the researchers determined whether each person had an "intention" to lose weight (defined as whether the person was currently attempting to lose weight). Then in 1981 they again obtained weights of the subjects. The researchers limited their analysis to those without preexisting or current diseases and followed them from 1982 until 1999. They compared the mortality for those who intended to lose weight with those of the group who did not intend to lose and actually maintained a stable weight. Those who intended to lose weight and were successful at it had mortality almost twice as high as those without such intentions. At least in this study, maintaining stable weight without intention to lose was "associated" with much lower risk of death. The authors concluded, "Deliberate weight loss in overweight individuals without known co-morbidities may be hazardous in the long term."[17]

Efforts expended to get their weight down could also end up having detrimental effects. Exercise may be a mortality risk factor. Jim Fixx, the guru of long-distance running, died during one of his runs. Would he have died anyway? Probably so, but perhaps not just then or in exactly the same way. And he might have had his problem in a setting in which he could have been rescued and treated.

Not every fat guy who launches an exercise program will do it under close supervision following a rigorous physical exam. Although that is often advised, not everyone will obey all the rules, and following the rules will not guarantee protection against adverse, unexpected consequences. Some people surely will die as a result of exercise programs who would not have died merely from being heavy. It seems reasonable to guess that more will be saved by their exercise program than will die from it, but I know of no study that has shown that to be the case.

Dieting may be another mortality risk factor. Diets radically change food intake. And even with vitamin supplementation, some critical element may be missing from one's diet. Total fasting seems to be the only thing that works for some people. Even physician-recommended strategies, such as the currently fashionable low-carbohydrate diets, are attacked by dietitians and by other physicians as being serious risks to health. Apparently, even diets developed by and closely supervised by health professionals can be controversial. Some of them no doubt increase one's risk of a serious, even fatal, outcome.

A colleague of mine was urged to go on a diet high in fruit and vegetables. One afternoon, following a physical exam, he got a panicky call from his internist. His potassium level was nearly lethal. Bananas, known to be very high in potassium, were included as acceptable foods on his diet, and he was eating lots of them. Whether banana consumption or something else caused the high potassium test was never determined. He stopped eating so many bananas, and his potassium level returned to normal. Had the potassium level altered his heart rhythm so as to cause a fatal heart attack, his mortality might have resulted from an attempt at weight reduction.

Some people sleep poorly when they diet. They lie awake nights stressed by feelings of hunger (or by feelings of anger that they have chosen to give in to social conformity and pursue prettiness). The same colleague who almost died from bananas says he has driven his car off the road twice because he nodded off from sleep deprivation during a course of dieting. I have never seen any figures on automobile fatalities associated with dieting, but I suspect there must be some. Fatigue and distraction play a key role in accidents, not only in automobiles but elsewhere as well. Before we conclude that weight reduction reduces mortality risk in any particular individual, we need to understand what the effect will be on accidents.

The most critical element of the relation of weight reduction to mortality and morbidity is probably not physical, but mental. Depression is rampant in our society. It is a major cause of death, directly by suicide and as a contributing factor to accidents and perhaps to physical disease. It probably contributes to compulsive eating and to resultant weight increases.

Depression is a feeling of hopelessness that results from a belief that one is perpetually trapped in a life that is unbearably unpleasant and from which there is no escape. If there were ever a cause for such feelings, it would have to be from pursuit of a socially mandated goal for the fat to become thin. Some dieters surely have serious, clinical depression. Clinical depression is a real risk for suicide and other causes of death. The risks of death from depression induced by worry about weight may not offset lowered death risk from weight reduction, but we cannot automatically conclude this. Dieting fat people may end up killing themselves in the process of trying to preserve their lives.

IS LIVING LONGER ALWAYS A GOOD OUTCOME?

All of these factual issues about weight and mortality may be a bit beside the point. The assumption that anything that allows one to live longer must be good is a remarkably naive one. Physicians of the 1960s held that whatever preserves life must be good, but that silliness was challenged by tragic medical cases such as that of Karen Quinlan, the young woman we met in the introduction to this book who apparently overdosed on tranquilizers and alcohol and was left for 10 years in a persistent vegetative state. We have learned from that example and thousands of others that there is more to life than merely extending days or months or years. Life exists in quality as well as quantity.

Sophisticated health planners now have a device for combining the amount of life one can expect from a treatment with the quality of that life. For each possible treatment, they ask how many years one can be expected to live and compare that number to what would be expected if the treatment were not provided. They then ask what the quality of those years will be. The result is that the quantity of life can be adjusted for or "discounted" for the quality. These quality-adjusted life years often get referred to simply as QALYs.

Living for 10 years with severe arthritis might, for example, be considered living a life at 90 percent quality, which would then be counted as nine "quality-adjusted life years." Using these methods, living a year of life in a permanent coma might be considered zero quality or no quality-adjusted life years.

Before deciding whether years of expected life added from weight reduction are worth it, each individual has to make a kind of crude QALY calculation. It seems reasonable that we should think of someone's "ideal weight" as the weight that is expected to produce the greatest number of years adjusted for their quality. It would be a miraculous coincidence if, for every living human being, expected QALYs were the greatest when one's body mass index was exactly in the 18.5–25 range. Some people may maximize their QALYs with a BMI greater than 25 or lower than 18.5. If so, it is nothing short of medical imperialism for medical experts to claim that weights in this range are ideal.

When it comes to a diet, if the number of suitably discounted, quality-adjusted life years added more than offsets the reduction in quality, then the diet is worth it. That individual is *overweight*. If, however, the number of years expected is offset by a reduction in quality of the years remaining, then what the NIH bureaucrats and other so-called health experts are offering when they publish guidelines for weight is an offer that any rational person ought to refuse. We are worse off (in QALY terms) if we are thinner. We are not overweight after all. We may be unfortunate souls who are fat, but at exactly the right weight. It would surely be irrational to try to lose weight if, by doing so, we reduced rather than increased the expected number of years (adjusted for quality) that we could live.

The Supposed Risk to Health

The drafters of the government standards may actually have something a bit different in mind, something a bit more sophisticated than the naive belief that we will always be better off if we live longer, no matter how miserable we are during those years. They may believe that even if we do not die, we will have more health problems if we are fatter. We may have an increased risk of morbidity (of disease, discomfort, and pain) resulting from our fatness that they feel would be lessened if we dropped down a bit.

Again, they may be right. It is not implausible to assume that various diseases and discomforts are related to weight. Reliable evidence exists showing an increase in diabetes, asthma, and arthritis in fat people.[18] The real questions, however, are whether the extra pounds cause these problems and whether we would be better off without them.

Fat and Disease: Does Being Heavy Increase Our Risk of Disease and Discomfort?

The evidence is mounting that various diseases are associated with higher body mass indices. Another recently published study, also in the *Journal of the American Medical Association*, shows that people who are "overweight" or obese (that is, a BMI of over 25) are generally at increased risk of adult-onset diabetes, gallbladder disease, coronary heart disease, high blood pressure, and high blood cholesterol level.[19] The NIH report also mentions stroke, osteoarthritis, certain cancers, problems in women's reproductive health, and psychosocial problems. This does not mean every fat person will get these diseases, but generally the odds are increased.

There are actually some oddities in the data suggesting that greater weight is not a disadvantage. Most physicians are not likely to emphasize these. For instance, among men, those considered overweight but not obese (i.e., those with a BMI of 25–30) actually have no increase in risk of coronary heart disease. Even more strange, the more severely obese older men (those over 55 with a BMI of more than 35) have no increased risk of high blood cholesterol level. (They actually had a lower risk, but the difference was not significant.) Among older women, the same result was found, but only for those with a BMI greater than 40. What this means is that these investigators found that fat people were at increased risk for many conditions generally thought to be bad, but not necessarily for all such conditions. There is even a hint that maybe some fat people may be at a lower risk for some disease-causing conditions.

This, of course, raises questions about whether these researchers are justified in calling fat people overweight. It rests on their judgment that one is more likely to have these disease conditions if one is fat, as well as their judgment that these conditions are bad. They believe fat people are better off enduring whatever it takes to lower their weight.

These authors, in comparison with the ones mentioned earlier, at least have the scientific integrity to say that these conditions are "associated" with being fat rather than that they are "attributed" to it. But even if the weight really does cause these diseases, it is not a fact that one is better off without them; it is a value judgment. It may also be that even though lowering weight really reduces the risk of these conditions, it also causes some offsetting kind of harm—some bodily trauma from the stress of the dieting, for instance, or some mental stress that is worse than the conditions one is trying to eliminate.

The real question then is whether these conditions and the diseases they presumably cause are bad enough that people would be better off eliminating the fat if they could. Here we are talking not only about serious chronic diseases, but also arthritis and other joint problems, sore heel tissue (plantar fasciitis), and countless other problems that are, by common stereotype, attributed to being fat. We could include the slower running speed and loss of agility attributed to fatness by sports team coaches who make a point of telling their athletes that they will perform better if they lose some weight.

The bottom line seems to be that it is probably wise to assume that being fat increases your risk of death and disease, but the story is complicated. The relation does not hold for all age groups and races, and some common factor may be causing risk for both fatness and disease. Even if we assume that these predictions of better body function for lower BMI people are true, the real question is whether we are better off lighter with our performance enhanced and our disease risk lower.

DO PEOPLE FEEL BETTER WITHOUT DISEASE?

This is one thing that smokers understand very well. No conscious, mentally competent adult smoker today is unaware that smoking increases (not just "is associated with") risks of mortality and morbidity. Still, many decide they are better off smoking and risking disease than if they are not smoking. That is a sad position for them to be in, but it may be an accurate assessment of their fate. Although I am fortunate never to have smoked and believe that everyone has the right to be informed about its dangers, I cannot honestly know whether everyone who continues to smoke is acting irrationally. Some would surely be better off if they quit. Maybe most would be. But deciding whether one is better off stopping requires a terribly difficult and subtle calculation, one that faceless medical scientists, who do not know the individuals involved and the agony they suffer trying to stop smoking, are in no position to decide.

Or consider the predicament of fat athletes. If the coach believes (even correctly) that athletes would do better at their chosen contests if they were thinner, it should be obvious that the question for the athlete is whether he or she is better off thin and agile, thus pleasing the coach, or fat, happy, and no longer on the team. It should be equally obvious that this will depend not on some scientific study, but on how badly the athlete wants to continue playing his or her sport and how miserable he or she will be slimming down. It is surely not the province of the medical scientists to decide whether people should improve their well-being by spending their childhood and young adult years competing for a place on a sports team or sitting in a library reading a good book. At most, the message seems to be a hypothetical or a "conditional." "If you would like to increase slightly the chance of being a star athlete (or if you would like to please your coach), lose some weight."

But what about reducing risk of diabetes or heart disease or gallbladder attacks? These are real medical conditions that scientists are telling us may be associated with being fat. Even here the conclusion that it is correct to lose weight does not follow. In the first place, even in the most recent studies, the relation between being heavy and the risk factors for disease was often not statistically significant. Only for the fattest—those with a BMI greater than 40—was statistical significance suggested. For most medical science, showing a difference that is not statistically significant is not showing much at all.

The more critical question is whether, even if higher BMI index really does increase the risk of disease, it is necessarily better to reduce one's risk. Rational people will not do everything they possibly can to increase the chance that they will live as long as possible (even if they are utterly miserable or unconscious while they live). Likewise, rational people will not lead lives that pursue elimination of every possible disease risk. The famous social philosopher and compiler of the Great Books of the Western World series, Mortimer Adler, was quoted as giving advice about success and happiness at his 80th birthday party. He advised, "Never exercise—as for dieting, eat only the most delicious calories."[20] He died at 98.

DOES ATTEMPTING WEIGHT LOSS HELP?

It is irrational to attempt to lose weight when, on balance, we have greater well-being fat and free of stress. The NIH fat police who tell us that over half the American population is overweight seem to believe that these people would be better off losing weight and that they fail to do so only because they are ignorant of the harm from being fat or lack the willpower to change. It seems much more plausible that the 150–200 million Americans who are labeled overweight or obese are fat because they are rational; they maximize their well-being at the weight that doesn't please the medical evangelists who would like to convert people to the new religion of slimness.

We may, in fact, harm our health as well as our well-being by repeated attempts to lose weight. That is suggested by one recent study. It should give the compulsive dieter pause. A group led by Linda Bacon, a nutritionist at the University of California–Davis, studied a group of 78 white, obese, female chronic dieters, aged 30 to 45. The women were given six months of weekly group intervention that was followed by an additional six months of monthly aftercare group support. One group of women was given a diet program; a second group was instructed in what was called a "health-at-every-size program." The health-at-every-size program emphasized body acceptance, eating behavior, nutrition, activity, and social support. According to the published study, in this program the focus was on enhancing body acceptance and self-acceptance. "The participants were supported in leading as full a life as possible, regardless of BMI."[21]

The small size and short duration of the study made it impossible to measure impact on mortality, but the researchers found that on many health-related variables, the health-at-every-size group made and sustained improvements whereas the diet group initially lost weight and improved on many variables, but relapsed so that little improvement was sustained. The health-at-every-size group sustained improvements in total cholesterol, LDL cholesterol, systolic blood pressure, depression, and self-esteem. The researchers concluded, "Encouraging size acceptance, a reduction in dieting, and a heightened awareness of and response to body signals appears to be effective in supporting improved health risk indicators for obese, female chronic dieters."[22]

Conclusion

So, are fat people overweight? Some undoubtedly are. That means they would not only live longer or lower their disease risk if they were skinnier, but they would also feel better and predictably add to their quality-adjusted life years (not just live longer and avoid disease).

Thus, some fat people may be overweight, but I suspect most are not. When the federal fatness authorities publish guidelines urging us to get below the mythical BMI of 25, they make terribly implausible assumptions. They believe that just because people below that cutoff line live longer and have less disease, the rest of us would get the same results if only we were rational enough to diet and exercise. And they assume that if people lived longer and had less disease, they would lead better lives. In short, they believe that 54.9 percent of the American public (not to mention countless other millions throughout the world) are too stupid, too stubborn, or too irrational to do what is good for themselves even in the face of hard evidence.

I suspect that people are not that dumb. I suspect that the millions who have tried to diet to the point of torture, pain, alienation, and agony are rational enough to figure out that even if getting their bodies down to some magical index level turned out really to increase their longevity and decrease their risk of disease, they would still be better off being somewhat heavier. The rational among us understand that there is more to life than living as long as possible. There is more to life than reducing disease risk to an absolute minimum. Living life at maximum quality *will* sometimes mean lowering weight below what provides maximum immediate gustatory satisfaction, but it also is likely to mean reaching some compromise with the federal government's BMI standard. Many who are fat by that standard simply are not overweight. They weigh exactly what, for them, is the best possible compromise. They are at their ideal weight, even if that ideal fails the tests for mortality, morbidity, and prettiness. Those people are fat, but not overweight. Many people are fat because they are rational.

| Universal but Varied Health Insurance

Only Separate Is Equal

Although the Clinton version of a universal health insurance plan collapsed in the political chaos of 1994, many Americans remain committed to some version of universal health coverage. Although new interest in health insurance seems to be emerging, and no viable proposal for universal health insurance has surfaced in America since those days, I will in this chapter use the Clinton plan as an example. Whether that coverage be a health service, such as Britain's, or an insurance coverage, such as Canada's or Germany's, the imperative to bring the United States up to the minimally decent standard of the rest of the developed world is strong.

The idea that dominates the "new medicine" is that deciding what counts as beneficial health care is fundamentally not a scientific matter, but rather a question of value judgments. This insight has radical implications for health insurance. In the era of modern medicine, the assumption was that experts could pick which medical services deserved to be included in a health insurance package on some objective, scientific basis. The treatments that were "medically indicated" were covered. The common insurance phrase is that health insurance covers what is "medically necessary." If it turns out that no treatments are medically necessary (as long as one is willing to pay the consequences), this standard for deciding what is covered is meaningless.

Is Physician-Assisted Suicide Medically Necessary?

Think of the dilemma raised by the legalization of physician-assisted suicide in Oregon. Physicians can now prescribe a lethal dose of barbiturates for certain terminally ill patients who have concluded they would be better off dead. They must be certified terminal and mentally capable of making an adequately informed decision. Their condition must be confirmed by a second physician. But once certified, a lethal prescription can be written by the physician.

How is an insurance company supposed to handle such situations? If their standard is that they will cover "medically necessary" treatments, how will they decide whether immediate death by actively taking a lethal drug qualifies. Some doctors, as well as some patients, will obviously find this particular "treatment" unacceptable. They may find it immoral, or they may simply decide they are not ready to die this way. For them, the prescription is not necessary; it is not even tolerable. For others, however, this may seem like the right choice. Their desire to die by taking a suicide drug may even be so strong that they say it is "necessary." Saying that it is "medically necessary," however, is odd to say the least. It may be psychologically necessary, but adding the adjective "medical" seems to do nothing to the concept of necessity. Surely, a physician's concurrence that suicide is urgently needed doesn't add anything to the judgment. An insurance company asked to fund this drug will face a problem.

The problem arises not only for the obviously value-loaded treatments such as abortion, cosmetic surgery, and physician assisted suicide. It arises for literally every medical treatment that could be imagined. Deciding to fund antihistamines for chronic allergy requires a value judgment that the symptoms that can be treated will respond in a high enough proportion of cases and their relief will be valuable enough to justify the expenditure of the community's resources. This, in turn, requires a comparison with all the other things the community of people who are part of that insurance pool might be able to do with the funds that could be spent on antihistamines.

Exactly the same point can be made about literally every service that health-care systems can offer. Surely, not every possible treatment that some subscriber believes offers benefit will be covered. Some of them—such as life-support for the permanently vegetative patient—are considered of no value whatsoever by a large majority of subscribers. Some of them offer such a small benefit at such a large cost that the only rational thing for subscribers to do is to demand that their premiums not be spent for these tiny benefits. When one realizes that the same treatments that are considered trivial by most subscribers may be crucial to a small minority, the idea that doctors (and other experts) can know what is best begins to pose very significant problems for the planning of health insurance. This chapter explores the implications for health insurance of the postmodern realization that deciding that a treatment is beneficial is always a value judgment. It argues that any single list of universally covered medical services will turn out to be grossly unfair and irrational because it will necessarily reflect value judgments that match the ones who draw up the list, that is, the most powerful members of the society. The more alienated and oppressed—those who stand farthest from the mainstream—will be the ones who get coverage for services that least match their values. The project of this chapter is to set out the broad outline of what health insurance should look like in the postmodern world of the new medicine. Then in the following chapter I will make the case for the moral necessity of what might be called "separate but equal" insurance plans.

Disputes continue over whether a universal, single-payer coverage would be governmental (whether it is a health service or insurance) or would, in a more typically American approach, rely on private insurance coverage. The Clinton plan, for example, would have developed administrative tasks to keep the private insurance industry employed. Whichever form the universal coverage might take, the appeal of universal coverage remains strong. It reflects egalitarian moral commitments that are deeply rooted in the American ethos no matter how unsuccessful efforts have been to operationalize that ethos.

A moral subtheme that will be critical to the political and ethical success of any universal health coverage is whether the plan will involve what has come to be called a "single-payer" structure and, regardless of whether there are single or multiple payers, whether the coverage provided will be exactly the same for all persons. As Dan Beauchamp, an early and thoughtful advocate of single-payer systems has pointed out,[1] it is possible that a single payer that managed the setting of reimbursement schedules and determined which medical services were covered could work through many private or public administrators. In a sense, federally mandated Medicaid coverage involves many state government administrations, but it is, to some degree, the federal government that determines the coverage and pays the bill. Thus it is possible to have a single-payer system with multiple administrators.

Likewise, it is possible to have other variations within a single-payer system. There may be a single or multiple tiers of services. There may also be a single or multiple lists of covered services. Thus when we debate single versus multiple structures, we need to be clear about whether it is payers, administrators, tiers, or lists that are the focus.

It is commonly assumed that if we go to a universal, single-payer coverage, everyone will get the same coverage, the same package of services. In many plans, however, all that will be provided is a basic tier of services. This is in accord with the moral commitment to a "decent minimum" or adequate level of coverage.[2] The Clinton plan would have provided only some basic level of coverage. In an era of consciousness for the need for cost-worthy care,[3] no one is promising to deliver every imaginable health-care service as part of the universal coverage. People are not even promising to deliver all useful or beneficial services. Some services that will do good and may be highly desirable, at least in the eyes of some consumers of health care, simply will not be included. There is no plan in existence today, no matter how lavish, that will cover every imaginable desirable service. Likewise, no universal, single-payer plan will provide all such services.

Single Payers and the Right to Additional Tiers of Health Care

To many this poses the major moral and practical problem of whether to permit people who have the means to buy additional tiers of services, either out of pocket or by buying a second or third tier of insurance using private, discretionary income. Such additional tiers of health-care services appear to undercut the moral egalitarianism that drives the quest for universal, single-payer systems. However, in a nation as committed to individual liberty and self-determination as the United States, few people believe that a prohibition on additional privately purchased services will be tolerated. Even among those who have attempted to argue on moral grounds that giving everyone the same level of health insurance would be fairer, there are few who really believe that discretionary purchases of additional levels of care will be prohibited.[4]

Moreover, even among egalitarians, considerable moral doubt remains about whether a compulsory single level of coverage is required. Consider luxury medical services such as cosmetic surgery and private Freudian analysis. These do not seem absolutely morally necessary in a basic insurance package, yet, assuming there will be discretionary resources available to some citizens (as there surely would be in any developed society), it seems plausible that those who possess discretionary funds could spend them on luxuries as they see fit, even on morally suspect luxuries, such as football game tickets, beer, or television sets. Egalitarians may want to insist that people receive only their fair share of surplus resources and that surpluses be distributed only after all are living at a decent minimum, but the availability of some discretionary resources seems plausible in contemporary society.

Assuming we are to be permitted to spend our fair share of resources on frivolous luxuries, surely those individuals who value face-lifts and Freudian analysis should have as much right to their favorite luxuries as do those who decide to buy whatever dangerous, mind-corrupting luxuries that are currently legally available to them. As long as the discretionary resources one possesses amount to one's fair share (however that might be determined), the option to buy a second tier of luxury medical services is not only politically inevitable, it is probably also compatible with many more or less egalitarian theories of justice. A single-payer system is in all likelihood compatible with a toleration of some purchases of additional services not included in its basic list of covered services.

Multiple Lists and a Single Basic Tier

Egalitarians who accept this conclusion are often comforted by the assumption that, at least at the level of the basic tier of services, everyone in a system with universal coverage would have the same list of covered health-care services.

One of the least controversial components of the Clinton proposal for a national health-care plan was the assumption that everyone covered under the plan would get the same coverage. Even if people were permitted to go outside the system and buy additional services with discretionary income, at least for the basics, everyone would be treated equally because everyone would be entitled to the same services. Although there are perhaps good practical arguments why a single basic package of covered services would be efficient administratively, I think the time has come to question the moral foundations of what I will call the "single-list assumption." However efficient it is to administer such a single-list plan, I think it is inherently unfair. If everyone is entitled to the same list of services, then those who place high value on the services on the list will get the most benefit, whereas those who value other kinds of services (alternative medicine, for example) will get relatively less. Of course, the ones who will value the services on the list will be the ones closest to those who design the list—the powerful elite who control public policy. In the next chapter I will even suggest that the practical problems with a single list may turn out to be so great that the single-list idea will collapse on administrative and practical grounds as well as moral ones.

SEVENTEEN

Health Insurance

The Case for Multiple Lists

The Inevitably Normative Nature of Health Benefits

The claim is that, in the era of the new medicine, justice will require not only that health insurance be universal, but that different insurance packages will offer different services. Consumers of health insurance will have to be able to pick the package that includes the best mix of services for them. They may pick high-tech medical services rich with organ transplants and artificial organs, but correspondingly light on some other services—perhaps psychological counseling or nursing care. Or they may pick a plan with hospice services, but no experimental cancer chemotherapy. The project for this chapter is to make the moral case for this arrangement, the case that, rather than being unfair because the lists are different, such multiple lists are a moral necessity for a system to be equitable.

The argument begins with a conclusion of much postmodern or contemporary bioethics that is the central theme of this book. Although modern medicine often functioned as if good medicine were a matter of scientific fact, postmodern or contemporary medicine has as one of its core premises the claim that literally every medical choice involves some sort of normative judgment about what counts as a desirable or good outcome. Although medical science may be able to tell us what the predicted effects of an intervention will be and what the odds are of certain side effects, in principle, it cannot tell us whether the outcome is *worth* pursuing or whether the risks of the side effects are *worth* it. In fact, it cannot even tell us whether an effect is an intended one or an unintended one, a side effect or a desired one. This is true not only with regard to morally controversial choices over abortion, sterilization, and termination of treatment; it is true of every decision made in medicine. Thus, in principle, no list of appropriate treatments for specified conditions can ever be prepared in the absence of evaluative judgments about whether the effects will be good or bad and, in either case, how good or how bad.

ARE NORMATIVE JUDGMENTS IN MEDICINE OBJECTIVE?

This observation has forced many people to conclude that all medical judgments are necessarily subjective. As we first saw in chapter 3, for some theories of value (what philosophers call *axiology*), the good is a function of what individual subjects prefer or what provides satisfaction of desires. According to these theories, deciding whether a treatment is good or bad medicine is inherently subjective. It is literally impossible to know whether the treatment will be labeled as good or bad without consulting some subject. Normally, the relevant subject is taken to be the patient or valid surrogate for the patient.

However, other theories of the good hold that objective lists of good and bad outcomes can be established.[1] According to this view, there is objectivity behind decisions about whether the outcome of a medical intervention is good or bad. A medical outcome really is "good" or "bad" regardless of the subjective preferences or desires of the patient (or physician). For our purposes, however, the critical element is that even with an objective theory of the good, it is not medical expertise that gives one the ability to know authoritatively which outcomes are good and which bad. That power rests only with experts in axiology (objective values), and in a secular pluralistic world, we have no ready means available for identifying who those experts are.

Thus, no definitive authority exists for generating lists of treatments that produce good outcomes or bad outcomes, and no authority exists for telling how good or how bad these outcomes will be. This is true regardless of whether one holds that judgments about the value of specific medical services are subjective or objective in character.

THE IMPLICATIONS FOR GENERATING
LISTS OF INSURED MEDICAL TREATMENTS

Thus, labeling a health service as beneficial always involves a normative judgment, and we have no obvious, accessible authority for deciding which services are valuable and which are not. One possible response would be to draw up a list of medical services that are desired, preferred, or thought to be objectively good by the majority of people or by a consensus of the population. It is hard to imagine, however, why one would want to try to generate such a majoritarian or consensus list. The most that one could say for this approach is that it would be easy to administer. Although that might count as a plus, it can also be the source of both unfairness and inefficiency. It would, at best, reflect the value judgments of the majority of the population, leaving those who do not share the majority values out in the cold.

It seems clear that no consensus exists over such a list. There are likely to be serious moral disputes about which services should go on the list. Some feminists groups would surely argue that abortion is a necessary medical service of immeasurable value, whereas some males and postmenopausal females would see little if any value in it for them and those in the pro-life camp would consider such interventions a terrible wrong. Some pro-life advocates would likely protest even to the point of violence to ensure that their insurance contributions or tax dollars did not go for this evil. Others would challenge the moral legitimacy of including aggressive cancer surgery, hospice care, liver transplants for alcoholics, circumcision, blood transfusions, or (in the case of Christian Scientists) virtually any medical interventions. Some would be angered that their insurance dollars were spent on other people's use of chiropractors or psychiatrists or whatever kinds of medical services they considered offensive, whereas others who see these services are crucial would be angered if they were omitted from the list of covered services.

Even for those treatments or procedures about which there is no open moral controversy, different people in different subcultures will evaluate the benefits very differently. Some will give high priority to the mental comfort from yearly mammograms for 40-year-old women, whereas others would consider that benefit too trivial to justify the monetary cost and the radiation risks. Some would give high priority to battles to preserve the lives of patients with metastatic cancer, whereas others would consider palliation a more appropriate investment.

Any attempt to force a universal insurance system to generate a single list of basic services will be divisive at best and grossly unjust at worst. It will be inefficient as well as unfair. Some treatments on any conceivable basic list will be so unattractive to some people that they will decline the service even if it is offered on a fully funded basis. In this case, these persons will be treated unfairly, even if no money is spent. They would be contributing insurance premiums or tax dollars to fund a list of services some of which they find to be of absolutely no value or even immoral.

More importantly, some people will face situations in which they view the services offered to them to be trivial and only of marginal value though very expensive. The person who has a slight preference for expensive, aggressive chemotherapy over a hospice program is likely to accept it if faced with a forced choice of accepting or declining the offer. Once he or she has contributed to the funding of the service, there is no self-interested reason to decline it. The only reason to decline would be altruism (that is, to save resources so others can benefit). This person will predictably get very little benefit from the funded service, whereas a medically identical patient who has a very strong desire for aggressive chemotherapy will receive much more value.

Any single list of covered services will be inefficient in this sense. People will be offered and often will accept services that are fully insured but for which they have only modest desires. If given a choice, they might well have had a much stronger preference for some other service that did not make the list. Even if there is a co-payment, the inefficiency will remain. Anyone for whom the marginal value of the listed service exceeds the co-payment will accept it.

Any single list of basic services that is part of a universal insurance system will appeal to some people's system of beliefs and values more than it will appeal to others. The closer one is religiously, culturally, and normatively to the makers of the list—that is, the closer one is to the center of power—the more value one will get from the list of covered services. Conversely, the more marginal one's system of belief and value, the less value one will get from the list of services covered.

In a modestly egalitarian world, the moral intuition that drives the quest for a single-payer universal health insurance system is usually some sense of fairness—the notion that it is unfair that people who are members of the same moral community get very different levels of opportunity to derive benefit from their health-care system. We tend to believe that people who are equally ill with the same disease should be treated equally, at least with regard to the basics. Yet, if equality is related to opportunities to obtain benefit, any single list of basic covered services cannot provide equal treatment. Such a list will give those closest to the list makers the most value they could get from the funds invested in health care. They will get exactly the services that they would buy if they were purchasing with similar funding on the open market. On the other hand, those furthest from the center of power will get, for the same premium, a list of services that does not appeal to them nearly as much, and hence is of much less value to them. They would, if they had a choice, prefer a different package of services.

Now we might be inclined to say that it is merely unfortunate that not everyone values the services offered in a single-list basic health-care plan in the same way. After all, even egalitarians do not insist that social programs must satisfy everyone equally or produce the same amount of happiness in all people. That would hold the program hostage to the people with the most lavish tastes, the ones most difficult to satisfy. All that egalitarians press for is access to equal levels of resources for people similarly situated.[2]

In the case of a universal, single-payer health-care system, it seems the reasonable and appropriate goal should be to give everyone access to benefits that the average consumer of health care could purchase for a fixed dollar amount. Thus, in our present health-care climate, a fixed premium of about $10,000 per family per year would probably constitute a decent basic level of coverage. There is no reason, however, that all must choose the same $10,000 package. To the contrary, doing so would be unfair as well as inefficient. Multiple lists of services should be available at this price.

For that fixed premium, the average consumer could buy an insurance package that would provide coverage similar to what is offered by private and public insurers. The premium could be adjusted upward in a wealthy society that had an expansive idea of the basic tier of services, downward in a society with more modest resources or a more minimalist view of a basic level of services.

Efficiency, Equity, and Multiple Lists

Is there any reason why members of a community who are provided with access to equal resources for health care necessarily must buy into exactly the same package of services? The standard response appeals to the efficiency of a single list. There would be no need to review claims to determine to which package of services the patient is entitled. There is also some appeal to the moral discomfort of caregivers who, if there were different lists, would have to treat medically identical patients differently even if they were lying in beds side by side on the same hospital floor.

The discomfort of caregivers probably is a result of the long-standing and justifiable discomfort at having to treat medically similar patients differently because some have equitable or even lavish insurance coverage whereas others are inequitably underinsured. Of course, caregivers ought to feel uncomfortable in those circumstances. But if people have chosen to invest in different, but equally funded, basic packages of health care, it is not at all clear that there is anything morally wrong with delivering different services to people who have different coverage. Moreover, the same problem will arise even if there were a single list of basic services. The Clinton plan and most others that have been proposed would permit the purchase of supplemental insurance and self-payment for additional tiers of services.[3] This would mean that two patients medically identical would be treated differently. Assuming that the purchase of the second tier of insurance was fair, they ought to be treated differently based on whether they have bought the supplemental coverage.

The inefficiency of multiple lists remains to be seen. Efficiency is normally measured in terms of the aggregate amount of good done per unit of investment. It is thus driven by utilitarianism. But I have argued that a single list will almost certainly mean that many people will buy many services that produce only marginal benefits for them. People whose understandings of the goal of medicine are not represented in the list drawn up will be faced with offers of covered services that are only marginally attractive to them. They would get much greater benefit if they were permitted to buy other services that are not in the basic list, but doing so will not be an option with a single list. Thus there are guaranteed inefficiencies in any single-list system. The number of quality-adjusted life years bought with a single list is certain to be smaller than with multiple lists. It is an open question whether the increases in utility from multiple lists will more than offset the expenses of tracking consumers to the proper list. Especially if there is single payer, with none of the confusions of fighting among private payers, there is reason to believe that the net benefit will be greater with multiple lists.

In fact, several existing government-funded health plans—including the insurance plans for government employees and those for Medicare enrollees—presently permit multiple lists of services. Government employees can choose from different insurance plans and Medicare enrollees can opt for HMO-type coverage if they choose. Here are models of single-payer systems with multiple lists that generate high satisfaction. These surely incorporate inefficiencies of private insurers, but they can serve as models for single-payer, multiple-list plans.

COVERAGE OF MORALLY
CONTROVERSIAL SERVICES

There is another dimension to any calculation of the efficiency of multiple lists. Some of the coverages in a single list will be extremely controversial. For example, a single list must either cover or exclude abortions under various circumstances. It seems a foregone conclusion that those opposed to abortion will be deeply offended if they are forced to contribute to an insurance fund that will be used to pay for abortions. There is every reason to believe that there will literally be rioting in the streets were that to happen. On the other hand, feminist and other pro-choice groups will be equally offended if abortion services are not included in their basic package, which also could easily lead to riots. Any single-list plan will have to take into account this type of dissatisfaction and potential social unrest in determining the amount of good that will result from the plan. Some compromise will certainly have to emerge.

Although no solution will satisfy all parties in a badly divided society, it seems that even the most militant pro-choice advocate should be willing to concede the offensiveness of forcing people to contribute to an insurance fund in which their money will be used to fund abortions. The least that can be done is to permit multiple insurance plans, some of which exclude services that are deeply offensive to people with particular moral convictions. Thus a Catholic Health Association list (administered by the government or by a private voluntary group if we retain a role for private insurers in a single-payer system) could exclude abortion, sterilization, artificial reproductive technologies, and other morally intolerable services. If their funding pool had payments equal to the other pools, then that pool would have monies left over for other valued services: natural family planning, more compassionate care for the dying, and any other services believed to be particularly fitting given the group's system of beliefs and values. If the result of exclusion of abortion were higher fertility, then the remaining funds would presumably be used for more child and maternal health services.

Certainly, the multiple-list approach will not completely satisfy the pro-life perspective any more than multiple lists through multiple payers does now. But it is hard to imagine a fairer solution or one that is more efficient in producing outcomes perceived as valuable and minimizing the social chaos that would result from forcing all persons into a single list.[4]

WOULD THE IDEA OF MULTIPLE LISTS
LEAD TO INFINITE REGRESSION?

There is another dimension to the concern about inefficiency. Although I have suggested multiple lists to meet the concerns of groups such as Catholics, feminists, Jehovah's Witnesses, and those who want unusually aggressive cancer treatment, given the number of variables at stake, it would be a mistake to assume that a single "Catholic" or "feminist" list would satisfy those identifying with these groups. Would there not therefore be subdivision and sub-subdivision to the point of infinite regress? Would we need to have a liberal Catholic list, a conservative one? An ultraliberal list and a moderately liberal one?

I think that is unlikely. The present federal health insurance presents a wide range of choices without succumbing to pressure to produce a different health-care plan for each government employee. Although there will certainly need to be more than one plan for Catholics, a relatively small number would probably satisfy the needs of Catholics (and others who hold similar values). Research on HMOs has suggested that groups numbering in the range of several thousand provide an adequate basis for efficient operation. It seems likely that one or two hundred lists would adequately cover the main value profiles in the United States. The result will not be exactly the coverage that each person would choose, but the lists would fit their values closely enough that people would not consider it worthwhile to study any further options. Probably the range of choices now available to government employees would be sufficient if they were standardized so that the payment, adjusted for age, were the same for each basic plan.

Residual Problems with Multiple Lists

Several residual problems would need to be addressed if a single-payer health plan retained multiple lists of covered services.

EMERGENCY SERVICES

Imagine some group that, if given the opportunity to create their own perfect list of desired health-care services, would exclude emergency room resuscitations as being expensive care that is likely to violate their sense of the goal of medicine. Perhaps some groups, such as Jehovah's Witnesses, would reject coverage only for certain emergency services such as blood transfusions.

For patients brought to the emergency room unconscious and without adequate surrogate decision makers, this would pose a problem. Their insurance would not cover the service, and yet there would likely be no way for the emergency room personnel to know this.

We presently rely on a presumption of consent for such emergency treatments at any point before the patient's objection can be known to the emergency room personnel. The alternative of insisting on actual consent for such treatments would have disastrous implications. Any multiple-list health insurance plan would have to cover certain services for which we presently presume consent in order to protect institutions from delivering unfunded care or, worse yet, having an incentive to fail to deliver such services. Any procedures that can presently be delivered under a presumption of consent would probably have to be included in all packages under a multiple-list plan.

SERVICES FOR THE PROTECTION OF OTHERS

Likewise, some medical services are mandatory because they protect third parties. Immunizations, quarantine, and some other services are presently required in order to protect the health of others. Such services would also have to be a mandatory part of coverage of all plans.

There are good reasons to argue that many services thought to be necessary to protect the public health (such as many immunizations) really do not protect something called the "public." Immunizations, for instance, may protect primarily the recipient of the immunization and free-riders who have chosen not to be immunized.[5] Nevertheless, to the extent that there are treatments that serve the public interest, they would also be candidates for mandatory inclusion on all lists of covered services.

MINORS AND OTHER INCOMPETENTS

Closely related to the problem of medical treatments to protect third parties is the problem of protecting the welfare of children. Although competent adults have the right to refuse any medical treatment offered for their own good, surrogates have a more limited right to refuse treatment on behalf of their minor children and others who are not competent. We have already litigated the limits on such rights so that we know, for instance, that Jehovah's Witness parents do not have an unlimited right to refuse blood transfusions for their children and Christian Scientist parents have a duty to provide certain medical treatments. Any such services found to be mandatory would have to be included as mandatory coverage in any list of insured medical services.

Note here a crucial difference between health care and education. Public school systems could be seen as single plans that force parents with minority values to either accept a single public approach or self-fund with additional money some alternative private educational system. But there are two important points that challenge this analogy. First, increasingly public schools *are* permitting multiple-choice alternative educational systems for parents who want to choose open classrooms or other innovations. More important, public education is by its nature a plan for minors. Just as society has a *parens patriae* obligation to make certain health care for minors mandatory, so also it has a similar obligation for the education of minors. The single option for education of minors is thus more defensible than a single concept of the good in health care for mentally competent adults. Certain goods are public goods: They cannot be obtained for some without obtaining them for all. Public security, roads, and the generation of knowledge (including medical knowledge) have this character. Most health care is not, in this sense, a public good. There is no necessary reason why if a service is funded for one group, it must be funded for everyone. Because people have very different ideas of the value of certain health-care services, they must be permitted to select the type of service that fits their sense of the good as long as it is within the budgetary constraints of a basic package of services—the $10,000 or so I have suggested.

HIGHLY PREDICTABLE RISKS

One of the more difficult problems for a multiple-list approach is how to handle conditions for which someone's risk is highly predictable. For instance, genetic diseases that are diagnosable prior to selection of a health plan would lead those who have determined that they are not at risk to select a plan that excludes coverage for these conditions. Caucasians might select lists that exclude sickle cell disease, Nordic gentiles could exclude Tay-Sachs disease, and so forth. If there were a single list, decision makers would have to choose whether to include or exclude various genetic diseases. It might be tempting to simply include them all, but some genetic conditions are likely to be perceived as too trivial to warrant coverage.

Probably the best solution is to figure out which genetic conditions that could be diagnosed prior to selecting an insurance plan would warrant coverage on a single list and then make that coverage mandatory on all lists. Undoubtedly there will be some unfairness of the sort that I have already argued will attend any single list: Those in power will pick genetic diseases based on their system of beliefs and values. The alternative for this special group of conditions, however, seems to be unacceptable. If persons were allowed to select lists that covered the diseases for which they were at risk and excluded those for which they were not, adverse selection would be so severe it would destroy the purpose of the insurance.

ADVERSE SELECTION BASED ON AGE

One of the more difficult problems of multiple lists is how to prevent adverse selection based on age. Because everyone knows that the elderly in general generate more health-care costs than the young, a group of young people could get together and create a list that excludes conditions of concern to the elderly, while being rich in services desired by the young. It would include good coverage for maternity services, well-baby clinics, fitness programs, and so forth, and omit services for senile dementias, arthritis, and other conditions of the elderly. The designers of the Clinton plan were well aware of this problem when they devised its original purchasing cooperatives approach. The solution proposed by the Clinton plan advocates would seem to work for multiple-list advocates as well.

The plan would collect a fixed dollar premium from every individual or family (my $10,000 figure, for example). That money would then be pooled by federal or state government agencies or whoever functioned as the single payer. The money could then be allocated to the funding pools for the different lists of covered services on an age-adjusted basis. For an elderly couple, for example, the funds contributed (from an employer, a government Medicare fund, or by self-pay) would be the same as for anyone else, but the transfer from the single payer to the various lists would be age adjusted so that the payment would be more or less than the amount collected based on the age-adjusted expected health-care expenditures. The allotment for an elderly person might be $18,000, that for 25-year-olds only $6,000. Because every person who survives to old age would pass through each stage, first experiencing periods when low payments were being made and later the provision of higher payments, the system would provide intergenerational fairness much as that for which Norman Daniels has argued.[6] If the age adjustment were properly calculated, designers of lists of services would have no incentive to attract the old or the young. The AARP-designed plan would include services attractive to the elderly, but the plan would get proportionally larger premiums for each member, canceling out any disadvantage of attracting many elderly people.

PUBLIC VERSUS PRIVATE MANAGEMENT
OF THE PLANS

I have mounted the case for multiple lists under a single payer, while keeping open the question of whether the management of the plan would be in public or private hands. There is no reason why a single-payer plan could not still rely on private groups—profit-making and nonprofit—to create and manage the lists. I would envision church groups, ethnic groups, and advocacy groups such as AARP playing some role at least in constructing the lists.

If, however, private, profit-making insurers continued to play a role, receiving their premiums from a single-payer purchasing agency, a problem would remain. Assuming the profit-making agency were allowed to keep as its profit any funds left over after the covered services were reimbursed, the agency would have an incentive to cover as little as possible. This would not be a serious problem if there were a perfect market because consumers would realize that for the $10,000 premium they could get more coverage elsewhere. However, the really clever profit-making insurance company would have an incentive to make its list look as generous as possible by including services that were cheap while looking very attractive. There would be an incentive for advertising and list construction that deceived consumers into believing they were getting more than they really were.

The most straightforward solution to this problem is to make the governmental single payer not only the payer but also the manager of the lists. If the Health Care Financing Administration (HCFA—the agency that presently administers Medicare) or some similar agency managed all the lists, their mandate would be to approve only those lists that actuarially were expected to break even. They would have no incentive to arrange one list to operate at a profit and another to operate at a loss. Every list would have a fund equaling: $10,000 adjusted for age multiplied by the number of subscribers. Perhaps private groups (the Catholic Health Association, Jehovah's Witnesses, National Organization of Women, or AARP) could submit lists for inclusion. Or they could submit lists (including all mandatory services) with some of their more marginal items rank-ordered so that they would be included only if the funds were expected to be able to cover the costs. But the final approval and management of such lists would fall to a body that had no stake in the lists' monetary performance.

Conclusion

The idea of a single-payer health system may be one whose time has come. Experience has shown that in other countries the single-payer system is far more fair and efficient than the current U.S. cacophony of plans. Movement toward such a single-payer system, however, should not be based on the assumption that a single-payer system is also a single-list system. When compared to a single payer managing a single list of covered services, it can be shown that the multiple-list approach is fairer in serving the interests of those furthest from the center of power. It may well also be more efficient in maximizing the benefits procured per dollar invested and in minimizing the offense of imposing a duty on some people to pay for services that they find deeply offensive morally.[7] A multiple-list plan avoids forcing people to participate in plans that are morally offensive to them while giving them a package of services that comes as close as possible to fitting their understanding of what the goals of medicine ought to be. Any insurance plan for a pluralistic society ought to provide multiple lists of basic covered services from which people may choose based on a universal entitlement to an equal age-adjusted level of resources.

EIGHTEEN

Why Hospice Care Should Not Be a Part of Ideal Health Care: I

The History of the Hospice

One important development in health care in the past few decades is the emergence of the hospice as an approach to caring for people with critical and terminal illness. Although it might seem odd, I want to suggest that the hospice should not be part of ideal health care. In this and the next chapter I will try to show why a hospice does not fit as part of postmodern medicine.

In the middle of the twentieth century in the height of what we have been calling the era of modern medicine, often the physician was committed to the value judgment that preserving life was the primary or even only goal of medicine. The patient was subject to all manner of torture for the purpose of striving to keep him or her alive—often without the patient's permission or even against the patient's will. A "death with dignity" movement emerged that fought the medical profession in hospital rooms, board meetings, and the courts to win the right for patients to accept or decline life-prolonging efforts.

From the perspective of the new medicine, the key is the realization that deciding what counts as good medical care for the critically or terminally ill—like what counts as good medical care anyplace else—cannot be determined by the judgment of the physician. Physicians may, at some point in history, believe that death is the great evil and is to be fought at all costs to the very end. Modern era physicians for a long time made that particular value judgment. Some are still stuck at that point, but it has not always been that way even in medicine. The Hippocratic doctor in ancient Greece was admonished not to accept the dying person as a new patient. That patient would end up dying, and it would look bad for the reputation of the physician. Darrel Amundsen (1978), the classicist who has long enlightened us on ancient Greek medicine, has argued that the duty to preserve life is a duty without classical roots.[1]

More basically, deciding what is the right goal for a dying patient is simply not part of what physicians should be expected to know about—at least not as physicians. It makes sense that Catholic physicians would turn to their religious tradition to understand the goals of life, the *telos* as that tradition frequently calls it. Only by consulting the theologians and teachers of that tradition and the basic sources of the tradition—scripture, reason, papal teachings, and councilor authority, in the case of Catholicism—can a believer, whether doctor or patient, know how one ought to do the work of dying. Whether death should be actively hastened, whether treatments can ethically be foregone as "extraordinary," whether pain should be suppressed or accepted as a character-building challenge, what spiritual preparation is appropriate before dying—all of these are critical questions for the dying Catholic, but they are not questions a physician can answer merely by his or her skills in medicine. In fact, they are not questions that even practicing Catholic physicians should be able to answer authoritatively (except in that rare case in which a physician is someone like an Edmund Pellegrino or a Dan Sulmasy—skilled physicians who are also, incidentally, masters of their religious tradition's theological doctrine). Even then, they can usefully provide spiritual counsel about the proper end of medicine for only that special group of patients who happen to share the theologically sophisticated physician's religious faith.

Similarly, Orthodox Jews should do their dying in a Talmudically prescribed way and should be counseled in those choices by someone skilled in that tradition's teachings—by a rabbi or someone with similar knowledge and training. Only in very special cases is a physician someone like Fred Rosner, who in addition to being a competent physician is schooled in the Talmudic tradition.

Likewise, there is a proper way for a Methodist or a Buddhist or a Marxist or a secular libertarian or a even Nazi to die, but the belief that the physician can be an all-purpose expert on knowing what are the right choices is a relic from the outdated modern era of medicine. Knowing all there is to know about the diagnosis, prognosis, and treatment options for the dying patient does not—in the postmodern era—tell us the right way to die.

The physician cannot be presumed to be the expert on making these choices. Only in the rarest of circumstances, when the physician is also skilled in the patient's system of beliefs and values, could the physician be expected to know how to advise the patient on choosing what is proper in the art of dying.

Some physicians eventually bought into the death with dignity perspective and decided that some medical interventions intended to prolong life were simply inappropriate. Unfortunately, in some cases they made this transition while remaining old-fashioned modern physicians. They continued believing that they somehow could know the right way for all their patients to die. In the extreme case, they sometimes came to the conclusion that keeping permanently vegetative patients alive with ventilators, blood-pressure regulation, and medically supplied nutrition and hydration served no purpose. Or they tried unilaterally to withdraw life support and force death on these patients against the patients' will.

By the 1990s physicians were often coming to the conclusion that providing some terminal illness life support was not serving the patient's best interest and was even contrary to the ideals of medical practice. They classified these treatments as "futile" and imposed nontreatment (that is, death) on patients unilaterally. The physician, in effect, ordered withholding or withdrawing of life support even in cases in which the patient or surrogate very much wanted treatment efforts to continue.[2] The modern physician still apparently believed that he or she could determine what was best for the patient even when it comes to deciding the time to die.

Postmodern medicine views these decisions as fundamentally not matters of medical fact. They are evaluative judgments that have to incorporate the personal beliefs and values of the patients and families involved in the decisions. That means that there is no such thing as a medically correct decision to transfer a patient to some form of terminal care involving something other than maximally aggressive life support. There is no "medically indicated" terminal care. The individual patient (or that patient's surrogate) will have to decide from a wide range of approaches to terminal care ranging from maximal life support efforts to various forms of "comfort care." The patient or patient-surrogate will have to decide exactly which treatments to provide and which to withhold.

Some very sick people will come to decide that certain treatments are not worth the candle. They will want to be kept comfortable, but not made the target of the full-court press. Many of these people will be good candidates to shift from a hospital or nursing home setting to an institution called a hospice. The issue for practicing the new medicine is how hospice care should be structured and financed once we realize that there is no such thing as medically correct care in these situations. Two medically identical patients who have decided to stop battling their cancer may choose somewhat different approaches to their care. One might want no curative treatment, but all approaches available for comfort—even if that involves palliative surgery, ventilator support for comfort, and medically supplied nutrition and hydration to prevent feelings of hunger and thirst. Another patient at the same stage of the same disease may prefer to back off on narcotic pain relief that can leave the patient in a stupor or forgo palliative surgery. Some patients may want to be on a ventilator to prevent conscious respiratory distress, whereas others would be willing to tolerate the distress or may choose "terminal sedation" to ease this discomfort. This means that proper terminal care will be infinitely nuanced with no two people choosing exactly the same treatment regimen. Any hospice care will have to accommodate this potentially extreme variation in what counts as good care in their cases.

Thus, hospice care will be a vital part of twenty-first-century life. That still does not mean, however, that it should be thought of as an important part of health care or should be covered by health insurance. Historically, hospice was not always seen that way.

Hospice in the Middle Ages

Hospices can trace their roots back at least to the medieval period when facilities existed throughout Europe. They were associated with monastic hermitages and convents and fulfilled a wide variety of needs. This was an era when the medical sphere was not sharply differentiated from other areas of life. The priest often served as physician. The needs of pilgrims and other travelers were met by hospices in religious institutions. They served as the equivalent of hotels, restaurants, places of spiritual retreat, orphanages, birthing centers, and leper colonies, as well as home for the sick and dying.

Sandol Stoddard,[3] the chronicler of the history of the hospice, notes there were 750 such facilities in England, but they also existed in major towns and cities throughout the continent. There were 40 in Paris, 30 in Florence. They appeared particularly at mountain passes and river crossings where pilgrims faced the greatest dangers. This diverse group of services—what Stoddard calls *hospitality*—were commingled in an era when there was no sharp division of labor separating medical from other caring roles. She traces a history back through the White Cross Knights of the eleventh century, to the Benedictines, the St. Bernard rescue dogs in the Alps, the hospice of

Turmanin in Syria in 475 CE, and a facility in Rome founded by Fabiola, a disciple of St. Jerome.[4] Whatever needs the traveler presented were on the agenda.

The Modern Hospice Movement

By the middle of the twentieth century medical care had become highly compartmentalized. Physicians were trained to focus narrowly on the health of the person in their care who could now be renamed as a patient—a name reserved for this specialized role as consumer of health-care services. In fact, often the health-care provider specialized further, concentrating on some small piece of this person called patient—on the liver or knee joint or esophagus. For the critically and terminally ill, the patient role was even further specialized. The patient was moved from the general practitioner or organ system specialist to the specialist in oncology, the radiologist, surgeon, chemotherapist, or hematologist. He or she was tucked away in specialized wards in specialized buildings in which medical care was the only object and cure was the passionate pursuit. When that effort failed, the health professionals involved were taught to believe that they had failed. More critically, they had no idea what to do but to keep trying more and more radical interventions hoping for a miracle in this most secular, rational of settings. The time had come to challenge this monomaniacal pursuit of cure.

CECILY SAUNDERS AND
ST. CHRISTOPHER'S HOSPICE

It is not surprising that the first challenger came from the nursing profession, the part of health care traditionally most comfortable with caring when cure is impossible. Moreover, it came very consistently from health-care professionals and groups with roots in the religious community.

Dame Cicely Saunders, called the "founder of the modern hospice movement,"[5] came to her calling from a deeply religious foundation. Entering training in 1941 at St. Thomas's Hospital, she underwent a religious conversion in 1945 at the age of 27. At first her interests were quite evangelical, but over the years she evolved into a high-church Anglo-Catholic.[6]

By 1948 she began working as a volunteer nurse at St. Luke's Hospital, one of the early homes for the terminally ill.[7] The pattern of hospitals named for Christian saints was already apparent. Saint Luke, known in Christianity as "the physician," is often associated with hospitals, especially those with a special mission toward the dying. It is here that she learned how to violate one of the norms of modern medicine. She risked overdosing her patients on narcotics by administering a "Brompton cocktail," a wonderfully rational drug mixture that includes a generous supply of morphine. She notes, however, that the St. Luke's version "omitted the cannabis and, I think, the cocaine."[8] This led her to medical school in the 1950s and then to St. Joseph's Hospice in October of 1958. The Irish Sisters of Charity who ran St. Joseph's were prepared to break still further with the modern medical tradition. She introduced a combination of morphine with alcohol and cocaine along with cyclizine, a drug that prevents nausea and motion sickness that has a calming effect. She adds, "having the time to sit and listen to a patient's story transformed the wards."[9]

In 1967 she carried this experience into the founding of St. Christopher's Hospice, which is generally considered the beginning of the modern hospice. It has become the model for hospices throughout the world. It challenged modern medicine's handling of death. This religious evangelist cum nurse cum physician cum saint pushed health care to new levels of imagination and compassion. More than health care was at stake. As she describes it, "This led to the concept of 'total pain,' which was presented as a complex of physical, emotion, social and spiritual elements. The whole experience for a patient includes anxiety, depression, and fear; concern for the family who will become bereaved; and often a need to find some meaning in the situation, some deeper reality in which to trust."[10]

Still her language was medicalized. This was a concept of "total pain." She provided care for "patients." The focus was still on pharmacological relief, albeit a much more enlightened understanding of what constituted relief. Escaping the clutches of the medical model was a very difficult task.

FLORENCE WALD AND CONNECTICUT HOSPICE

In the United States the hospice movement had its beginnings with another nurse, Florence Wald, who had served as the dean of Yale's School of Nursing and founded the Connecticut Hospice in 1974. She had the active support of clergyman Ed Dobihal and others in the community. Hospice was once again challenging traditional medicine. The goal was no longer to fight disease and death. In fact, it was no longer even medical in the usual sense. It was an effort to serve the whole person with religious, economic, social, artistic, and cultural needs, as well as medical. Although at first she began developing an interdisciplinary team at Yale, she soon found the medical setting too confining. Physicians were frightened to administer adequate pain medication. She later observed that the health-care setting and medical schools made it a hard struggle to establish humanistic care. When she visited St. Christopher's in England, she says, "I recognized the freedom they had in this autonomous institution to go about their business."[11] Nevertheless, the Connecticut program was instilled with the medical model. It was led by a nurse and dominated by medical concerns—pain relief, adequate sanitation, and control of symptoms. It was a nursing project even if it was nursing at its most enlightened.

THE GROWTH OF AMERICAN HOSPICES

Beginning in the mid-1970s the hospice idea caught on. It rode the wave of the death with dignity movement. For every patient who realized that fighting death with aggressive surgery, radiation, and chemotherapy was not the way to die, there was a person struggling to be liberated from the medical model. It was a person who didn't want his or her last days to be exclusively in the role of patient. It was a person who wanted the last stage of life to include a wide range of concerns: religious, familial, recreational, economic, legal, and social. In the next chapter I suggest an alternative to a hospice as part of high-quality health care.

NINETEEN

Why Hospice Care Should Not Be a Part of Ideal Health Care: II

Hospice in a Postmodern Era

It is obvious that the hospice movement has grown out of the medical model. It is health professionals—mainly nurses—who have been the leaders in the development of hospices. That has often led to choice of language and methods of procedure that are medical. We sometimes talk about the staff of hospices as "health-care providers." More critically, we talk about the lay participants in hospices as "patients." We do this even though much of what a hospice participant receives has nothing to do with health care as normally understood. The hospice participant receives companionship, help with housekeeping, and so forth. He or she is read to, joked with, prayed with, and cried with. In "inpatient" hospices, the participants might better be called "hospice residents." In home care, they remain residents in their own homes and might be called variously "owner," "resident," "participant," or some other label. Calling these persons "patients," however, categorizes them into the medical model.

The effect of medicalizing hospice is subtle, but important. If it is a medical organization, the type of staff that would come to mind first is health professionals—doctors, nurses, pharmacists, and social workers (perhaps with dietitians, chaplains, and others who are connected with medical care). Housekeepers, clergy who are not chaplains, lawyers, educators, artists, accountants, and architects—all of whom should be critical to providing integrated support to dying people—do not come to mind as readily. It is these nonmedical specialists who provide much of what dying people need. Medical care is only a minor part of hospice, just as it is a minor part in the rest of life. If we think in terms of the board of directors of the hospice, medicalizing the hospice will inevitably overweight the membership with medically oriented people. The budget is likely to be centered on health services and health professional staff.

If the hospice resident is to be thought of as a whole person going through a final stage of life, he or she should not be reduced merely to the patient role. The full range of needs and interests should be part of the hospice program. Legal concerns about wills, home ownership, and inheritance may get short shrift. So might architectural concerns about redesign of houses and recreational and artistic concerns. Hospice care, in short, is not a division of medical care focusing on the end of life; it is, or should be, an integrated program for services at a stage of life when needs can be great and many people from many professions can be of great help.

Why Hospice Care Is Not "Medically Indicated"

Based on this notion that a hospice program should focus in an integrated way on the total needs of the dying person and should not be thought of as merely a type of health care, we can't escape the conclusion: It is a mistake to medicalize hospice. When this is combined with the linguistic concerns raised in chapters 7–9 about the language of the new medicine, it should be obvious that hospice care is never "medically indicated." It is not "medically indicated" not only because deciding that hospice is appropriate is always a value judgment, but also because hospice care involves much more than medical care. Within the medical component, the choice of terminal care plans is inevitably subjective and necessarily determined by patient preferences. There is no "treatment of choice" for terminal illness. Rather, there is a set of services, some of which may turn out to be medical, that will turn out to fit the needs and interests of the dying person. Many of those services are simply not "treatments." Those needs and interests may turn out to be addressed best by volunteers (e.g., shoppers, readers, and housekeepers), chaplains and social workers, lawyers, accountants, architects, educators, artists, and musicians. Two examples help make the case.

Bill Monroe and the Nursing Home

I am a student of early American mountain music and its descendant called bluegrass. One person is credited with single-handedly creating bluegrass, and that is Bill Monroe—a recipient of the National Medal of the Arts. His band, the Blue Grass Boys, is the foundation for a unique American genre. He had his influence, in part, because he played so long—from the founding of the band in 1939 until shortly before his death in 1996. Playing well into his 80s, he survived major heart surgery to return to the road until a stroke silenced him.

Left aphasic in a nursing home in Springfield, Tennessee, he was reportedly quite depressed, as well he might be having spent his entire adult life on the road in a touring bus with his band, playing the music he loved with unequaled passion.

Although Monroe was the father of this music, other bands have been crisscrossing the country in touring buses for almost as long. Among them is the band of Mel Goins, who played briefly in Monroe's band (in 1958) before starting out with his brother, Ray, as the Goins Brothers. Illness forced Ray to leave the band in the early 1990s, but Mel Goins is still traveling with his group, now called Windy Mountain (after a famous old song he performed years ago).

Goins's bus was passing through Tennessee near the nursing home that was to be Bill Monroe's last place on earth. Goins decided he had to stop. Worried that he would be disturbing a very sick man and feeling uncomfortable in the medical setting, Goins cautiously approached, leaving the rest of the musicians in the bus for what was to be a brief stop.

What he found was a sad shadow of what was once the most powerful force in the field, a man who could not talk or walk or even gesture. As Goins told the story to a group of us gathered in the Blue Ridge Mountains for one of his performances, he just could not stand what he was seeing. He cautiously asked a nurse if it would be all right if he got his guitar. He knew he was treading on medical turf. Like the rest of us, he was unsure of himself when he entered a hospital or nursing home. We know we must play by the rules of the authorities who have strange attitudes about what we can or cannot do.

Some wise nurse said she thought it would be all right, so he went back to the bus and got his guitar. Like every long-term music professional in bluegrass music, he knew every song Bill Monroe had recorded, and Goins could reproduce the sound the way Monroe demanded it be played. With the first notes of the music Monroe owned, Goins saw a smile cross Monroe's face and his fingers tapping out the rhythm. Soon Mel Goins was back on the bus getting the rest of band, who held an impromptu concert at the nursing home. He described the obvious joy on the face of a very proud but now speechless man. Mel Goins had taken back the musician's turf from the health professionals. What he did was just common sense, humane compassion. Any dying man should be entitled to enjoy the music he invented. It didn't fit the nursing home's medical model, but it surely fit the style of dying of the father of bluegrass. What Mr. Monroe needed for his hospice was not physicians or even nurses; it was an old friend playing the music for which he had given his life.[1]

CASE 19.2

The Social Worker as a Saint

The second story is different; even more tragic. A young man in his late 20s lived in Washington DC. He was about to be just another victim of HIV dying another unspeakably tragic death. Again, it was not his disease that was the problem; it was his society. He was uninsured and essentially a foreigner to the health-care system, but that was not his problem. District of Columbia Medicaid would cover his medical costs, and adequate care was available, at least in theory. He was also poverty-stricken and alienated from a dysfunctional family. His father had not been part of the family in years. His sisters were living in the suburbs, desperately trying to escape a hopeless hellhole of a home they had left.

This young man was left deteriorating rapidly toward death in what was supposed to be the care of a mother who was a mentally ill drug addict. She was supposed to be feeding and nursing him, but would disappear for days at a time on drug binges.

He was left immobile, bedridden in a single room that was supposed to pass as their residence. The heat and electricity had long been disconnected because the bills were not paid. The windows had been broken out in a fight in the room. Now, in the middle of a cold winter, this man was at the mercy of a mother who, when she was present, was offended when members of a hospice team tried to come and help.

The hospice team tried to arrange for what would pass as friends to drop in on him to help with cleaning excrement from the bed and floor, washing bedding, and making sure that food was left within his reach. The mother would threaten the hospice workers when they appeared.

His need was obvious. The hospice social worker—twenty-something and petite—would climb the dark stairs of this room deep in the heart of the worst crime infested neighborhood of the city. It was routine for the hospice to provide nurses and social workers with an armed police escort, but she often made the trip alone because the police were afraid to come here.

She knew what this man needed—transfer to a nursing home or a residential facility such as the Whitman Walker Clinic, the last best hope for the hundreds of young, HIV-infected men without any place to turn. The problem was that—believe it or not—his mother had intimidated him into feeling guilty if he abandoned her. In addition, he knew he did not want to do his dying in a place that was his image of a nursing home—with elderly, immobile, mentally deteriorating patients.

The social worker's strategy was to convince him to visit Whitman Walker to see that it was not what he imagined. It was a place where people much like him could relax, receive good care, and die at peace. She thought she could get him to agree to move there if she could only get him to visit for a few hours. That meant a round-trip ambulance ride because he was in no condition to travel in a car or taxi.

The problem was that Medicaid would pay only for transport by ambulance for a life-threatening emergency or as a one-way trip to a nursing home. She asked the hospice to raise the money for what amounted to a round-trip taxi ride in an ambulance. Once she convinced the hospice to use a very small discretionary fund to pay for the ambulance, he made the trip and agreed to a permanent move, freeing him from what may be the worst living conditions I have ever heard a dying man have to suffer. That social worker understood that hospice care was something far greater than medical care.

These two cases show why hospice care is crucial during the last days of life. These two people—the world's greatest bluegrass musician and what was perhaps the world's most miserable person—both had desperate needs.

Their medical needs were manageable. Their emotional, social, and comfort needs were overwhelming. Medicaid does not have budgets for bluegrass bands or for taxi rides. It doesn't fund glaziers to repair broken windows or pay heating bills. It doesn't provide police to protect grown men from their mothers or from crime-infested neighborhoods.

In these two cases, dying people got what they needed. They got it because Mel Goins happened to be passing through and a saintly social worker persisted when mere mortals would have had every right to abandon their assignments. Only by liberating life in its final phase from the medical model can we hope that these relatively happy outcomes will be repeated.

How Medicalizing Hospice Care Distorts It

Medicalizing hospice care can distort it by letting the medical component dominate when nonmedical services may turn out to be more critical. Placing a hospice in a hospital or nursing home runs the serious risk that hospice will be overmedicalized. Medical institutions force on people—health professionals and laypeople alike—a set of behaviors and a style that is unique and alienating. Hospices almost have to be corrupted by these powerful influences.[2]

In Washington DC there were two hospices for many years—the Hospice of Washington, which is a subdivision of a nursing home called the Washington Home, and Hospice Care of DC, which began as an independent, freestanding hospice facility and has recently merged with other freestanding hospices in the Washington metropolitan area to form Capital Hospice, which serve the Washington DC metropolitan area.

I was the President of the Board of Hospice Care of DC when it was exploring possible mergers and considered merging with the Hospice of Washington. The Hospice of Washington was a very respectable, old organization with a great deal of integrity, but merger talks ran into a serious problem. The conversations about the model of care that would be provided by the hospice seemed inevitably shaped by the fact that Hospice of Washington was embedded in a nursing home and the staff and board were thinking in terms of nursing services. The hospice, which was supposedly committed to integrated services extending well beyond health-care services, was operating in a building and under the supervision of administrators and a board of directors that thought in health-care terms, not in terms of a dying person whose needs may extend well beyond the medical. It was not the world of bluegrass bands, taxis, and architectural redesign.

Placing a hospice in a nursing home, a hospital, or other medically oriented system provides what can be called "vertical integration." A vertically integrated health-care system (such as an HMO) can provide "cradle-to-grave" service that, at best, integrates the medical component of a person's needs throughout life. By contrast, freestanding hospice provides "horizontal integration." The focus is on the full range of needs of a person at a particular time of life—the time of dying. A freestanding hospice asks what is the set of services needed by a person—not a patient—at this time in the person's life. The staff and board should be just as concerned about all the nonmedical areas of the person's needs. They need bluegrass musicians and ambulance-taxis as much or more than physicians and nurses. They need artists, shoppers, companions, architects, and spiritual soul mates.

The merger to form Capital Hospice would provide another kind of integration. In the Washington metropolitan area, geographical integration can be problematic. A person living in suburban Fairfax County, Virginia, may receive her medical care in the District of Columbia, go to church in Montgomery County, Maryland, and participate in the museums and artistic venues in all these jurisdictions. If a good hospice needs to facilitate all of these contacts, a merger with the other freestanding hospices of the metropolitan area seems right. I was very pleased when it finally decided to merge with the other freestanding hospices rather than buying into the more geographically limited program under the aegis of a nursing home, even though the nursing home was one of great stature and quality.

A hospice program in a postmodern society must be much more than a health-care program for the dying. It must be a total program of integrated services, only one of which counts as health care. It is impossible for a doctor to know what is best for a *patient* even in the sphere of medical decisions. It is even more impossible for health-care professionals to know what is best for a dying *person* when one recognizes that the person's needs extend far beyond the medical.

Hospice Care and Health Insurance

This separation of hospice care from the medical model in the world of the new medicine will have implications about how hospice care ought to be funded. There has been great pressure to make sure that health insurance programs include a hospice option. Likewise, public health insurance such as Medicare has developed coverage for hospice services. The concept of hospice developed in this chapter has surprising implications for these funding commitments.

WHY HOSPICE SHOULD NOT BE PART OF HEALTH INSURANCE

If hospice should not be thought of as a part of health care, then it makes no sense for health insurance to cover it. If it does, it will be supervised by health insurance auditors—public and private—and would have to meet requirements that can be expected for medical benefits. In many jurisdictions, such as in the District of Columbia, any new expenditures of health-care dollars in public programs such as Medicaid must meet standards for a "certificate of need," or CON. In order to control costs, a health-care-oriented government agency has to approve of the new program. This way duplicate and unneeded facilities (such as extra hospital beds or CAT scanners) can be blocked so that taxpayers' health-care dollars are invested in a cost-worthy way.

This poses a problem for an organization such as a hospice. Many of its programs are not really "health-care" programs. In fact, if hospice benefits are measured by traditional health-care criteria, the program often can look like it is doing poorly. To take an absurd example, in a traditional health-care program, benefits might be measured by how long participants survive. By this standard, a hospice program is always a miserable failure; its patients die quickly. More problematically, many of the budget items in a good, integrated hospice may well be directed to personnel and other expenditures that do not have any effect on traditional health outcome measures. The expenditures for supervising volunteers, driving program participants to shopping, the library, or social events, and the costs for nonhealth-care professionals may have no impact on health-care outcome measures. This gives the bureaucrats evaluating CONs a good excuse to give a hospice low priority. Because the CON process is a very political one, a small independent hospice will be up against large corporate conglomerates that have an interest in preserving their market share for health-care dollars. Those health systems may run nursing homes, extended care facilities, and palliative care programs that are directly threatened by a freestanding hospice. It is easy pickings for the health system megacorporation to use its political clout to block a small hospice's CON. Because the personnel in the government agency responsible for the CON are often health-care professionals themselves, frequently moving back and forth between their government agency and the health-care industry, they tend to see decisions about need in terms that are sympathetic to the more traditional health-care institutions.

Hospices really don't have much of a chance. Because much of their program should really not be seen as health care in the first place, this is understandable. There is good reason to get hospices outside the health-care system. Even ideal health care should not include hospice. Hospice needs to be conceptualized in much broader, more integrated terms as a crucial part of the social system that meets important needs of the population for a wide range of services at an important phase of their lives. This is not properly thought of as health care; it is more-inclusive social service. Hospice needs to be more like the hospice of the medieval monastery, less like a well-run nursing home.

WHY HOSPICE SHOULD BE PART
OF SOCIAL SECURITY

This, of course, does not in any way imply that hospice services are not important or should not be funded. Hospices provide some of the most useful, compassionate, and humane support that could be imagined for some of our most vulnerable community members. In fact, hospice service should be available—at public expense—to anyone who chooses to use it. It simply should not be funded through health insurance. Not only does health insurance pose all of the problems we have just encountered, it also poses serious limits on access. Although the Medicare hospice benefit covers everyone eligible for Medicare—that is, virtually all elderly persons and certain persons with chronic disabilities—it excludes almost everyone under age 65. Medicaid covers some of the poor who are under that age, but it excludes many of the poor who are not capable of handling the bureaucratic requirements of the applications and paperwork.

The alternative is obvious. There should be a universal entitlement to hospice services adequately funded for all citizens and permanent residents of the United States. This could be an independent new program, but it would probably be much easier simply to attach it to Social Security. Virtually everyone participates in Social Security, at least to the point of having a number. A hospice benefit as part of Social Security would be analogous to other benefits in the program, such as a death benefit.

The advantage of placing a hospice benefit in Social Security rather than in health insurance is that it would be separated from the medical model. There would no longer be an incentive to rely exclusively on health professionals as the administrators and bureaucratic decision makers for hospice coverage the way medical insurance does. It would make it clearer that hospice is supposed to spend a significant portion of its budget and hire a significant portion of its staff to provide services having nothing really to do with health care. It would mean no more CON controversies, no more linking of hospice coverage to employee health insurance, and no more medicalizing of what is really a broad, integrated human service. Hospice should not even be part of ideal health care; it should be part of humane, compassionate care for the terminally ill that extends well beyond health care.

III

THE NEW MEDICINE AND THE NEW
MEDICAL SCIENCE

| Randomized Human Experimentation

The Modern Dilemma

Research medicine is another area that must undergo fundamental change in the era of the new medicine. In the modern era, medicine came to be dominated by what came to be called the "gold standard" of medical science, the randomized clinical trial. Because medical decisions were believed to be based on medical science, it seemed to stand to reason that good science could tell physicians which treatments were "medically indicated" or "treatments of choice." We have seen in chapters 8 and 9, however, that these notions are no longer meaningful in a world in which all medical choices involve value judgments. Now we need to see what the ethics of medical research is like in the new world of postmodern medicine.

It came to be a standard assumption of modern medical science that individual physicians and patients could not know which treatments were best simply by administering drugs and watching to see what would happen. No one could ever know whether the effect would have occurred anyway. If a drug were given to a sick patient and she got well, we still didn't know whether the drug was what made her well. In fact, it might just be that she would have recovered even sooner without the drug.

We couldn't even answer the question of whether the drug was making patients better by looking at a large group with some disease who took the drug and comparing them with another large group who seemed to have the same disease who did not take the drug. We came to recognize that some other factor might be determining who took the drug and who did not. For example, if wealthier people tended to be the ones taking the drug, their wealth might also have influenced their behavior in some other way that was really making them better—they might have a better diet, better education, more immediate access to physicians, or something like that.

The solution was the randomized clinical trial in which a large group who had some condition upon which physicians wanted to test a new drug was assigned randomly to get either the drug or some other treatment (either a previously standard treatment or a placebo designed in such a way that they could not know which compound they were receiving). Likewise, because the researchers themselves might be biased if they knew which treatment the various patients were receiving, the knowledge of which agent was also kept from the researchers. Because the knowledge of which compound was given to each patient was kept from both patients and researchers and the patients were assigned randomly to one or the other treatments, this was called a randomized, double-blind clinical trial. Only after the patients' results were recorded and classified did the researchers learn which treatment was which.

This posed a moral dilemma for doctors of the modern period, however. If the doctor believed one treatment was best for his or her patient, how could the physician intentionally let treatments be assigned at random so that patients would be exposed to anything less than the best treatment?

The Classic Version of the Dilemma

The Hippocratic physician was supposed to be loyal to his or her patient. This requires choosing only the therapy that the physician believes is best for the patient. How can physicians choose only the treatments they think are best for their patients and still recruit them to be randomized, thus condemning them to a chance they will receive a treatment that is less beneficial or even a useless placebo?

Physicians of the modern period thought they had an answer to this dilemma, at least in some cases. We can call it the "standard answer." We shall see that the standard answer actually turns out to fail to solve the problem. In fact, the problem cannot be solved until we shift to the premise of postmodern medicine—the premise that deciding what is the best treatment requires the evaluative judgments of the individual patient.

THE STANDARD ANSWER: IN TWO PARTS

The standard answer of the modern period comes in two parts. The first relied on the insight that in certain situations a clinician may have two or more options for treating a patient and may be indifferent or ambivalent between the options. The second addresses the fact that even though one physician may be ambivalent between treatment options, his or her colleagues may have a decided preference. Or conversely, the clinical community may be ambivalent between two treatment options even though a particular clinician has a decided preference.

The Standard Answer, Part I: Clinicians May Be Ambivalent between Options

Consider first the situation in which a patient is under the care of a physician in the modern era and that physician, faced with the task of choosing a treatment for the patient, considers two options and can't really decide which is better.

The Role of Physician Ambivalence

That clinician may have no basis for choosing between two standard therapies, between a standard therapy and an experimental one, or between an untried therapy and a placebo. If the clinician is really torn between the two options, he or she would presumably (metaphorically) have to flip a coin. The standard defense of the randomized clinical trial in the modern era holds that the clinician may, if uncertain which of two treatment options is preferable, justifiably offer the patient the opportunity to be randomly assigned to one of the options. This basis for justifying randomization is sometimes referred to as the "uncertainty principle."[1]

It is rare, however, for a clinician to be absolutely uncertain or indifferent between two treatment options. Such ambivalence is also rare if one is testing a new treatment for a condition that is treated inadequately with existing therapies. For an experimental treatment to be worth testing, there must be some reason to hope it may be better than the standard treatment. There must be some theoretical insight, some animal data, or some anecdotal evidence from other patients suggesting a reason why the new treatment is plausibly preferable. But if there are reasons to believe that the new treatment is attractive, it is not always easy to remain indifferent when comparing it with standard treatment, especially if that treatment is not very effective. If the new treatment offers many potential benefits and no disadvantages, then the clinician should not be ambivalent. To be legitimately ambivalent between a promising experimental therapy and a not-very-effective standard one, there must also be fear that the experimental treatment may have a downside—an unexpected side effect, perhaps even a lethal effect.

In my service on institutional review boards (IRBs) and data safety and monitoring boards (DSMBs), I have seen investigators desperately attempting to sell the review board on the potential advantages of the experimental treatment, only to be challenged with the question, then how can you justify randomizing patients and exposing them to the risk of getting the old, less attractive standard therapy? The investigator usually at this point makes a rapid discovery of the potential risks that might offset the potential advantages of the experimental agent.

In order to justify randomizing against a placebo, two things must be true: (1) There must be legitimate doubt whether the experimental agent is better or worse than the placebo (i.e., worse than doing nothing), and (2) there must be no other therapy—no standard therapy—that seems clearly better than *either* the placebo or the experimental agent. If clinicians are legitimately ambivalent between two treatment options, it is usually claimed they are morally justified in recruiting their patients into a randomized trial. When these conditions obtain, the clinician is at a position I have called the *indifference point.*[2]

Others, going back to the Harvard lawyer Charles Fried's analysis, have used the term *equipoise* to refer to this condition.[3] The physician is "equally poised" between the options. Because the situation is one in which the patient's physician is ambivalent between two treatment options, it could be called *individual clinician equipoise.*

Two Problems with Physician Ambivalence

There are, however, two problems with the first part of the standard analysis: Absolute indifference is rare, and individual clinicians may have idiosyncratic indifference.

1. Absolute Indifference Is Rare. First, as we have noted, individual physicians are rarely, if ever, absolutely indifferent between two treatment options. They will almost always have some basis in experience, in the scientific literature, or in their risk-taking inclinations, to have at least a slight preference for one or another of the available options.

It is here that most physicians and patients are willing to make a modest departure from strict Hippocratic ethics.[4] Given that other patients and society in general may have a crucial interest in determining scientific knowledge accurately, they will accept that it is moral, with proper permission of the potential research subject (or a valid surrogate), to ask the individual to agree to sacrifice his or her interest at least slightly if such sacrifice is necessary to contribute to important scientific knowledge.

Consider the situation in which a medical researcher wants to impose a small risk on a normal subject (such as drawing a small amount of blood) or ask a patient to receive a treatment that has an expected net benefit that is slightly less than the standard treatment (such as accepting a risk of receiving a placebo rather than aspirin for a mild headache[5]). Most people would agree that it would be acceptable morally for a physician to ask the potential subject to agree to accept the incremental risk for the good of science. They agree it is acceptable even though making such a request is incompatible with the Hippocratic ethic. As long as the sacrifice that is requested is modest and the patient gives an adequately informed consent, such requests seem perfectly acceptable.[6] We can say that all that is needed is "approximate indifference" or a small enough marginal risk that the subject is willing to make the sacrifice for the good of science.

Hence, if the physician is approximately indifferent between the two treatment arms, we seem to have satisfied a necessary condition for ethical randomization. Throughout the rest of this chapter and the next, when I speak of indifference, I shall assume the qualification that the indifference does not need to be complete, that *approximate indifference* is sufficient to justify a randomization or other research intervention in which a subject is exposed to a procedure that is not for the subject's benefit.[7] As long as the expected benefit/harm profile of the intervention is approximately as attractive as the alternative and there is an adequate consent, the research intervention will be taken to be justified.[8]

2. *Individual Clinicians May Have Idiosyncratic Indifference.* In the world of the new medicine, there is a more serious problem: Individual clinicians may be idiosyncratic in their comparisons of the two interventions to be randomized. The individual clinician may be indifferent even though none of her colleagues sees it the same way. The clinician may not have access to all the data. She may have experience only with a small, biased sample of patients. Most critically, she may have unusual values that lead to unusual evaluations of the anticipated benefits and harms of the two treatments.

CASE 20.1

Physician Preferences about Megadose Vitamins

I served on the data safety and monitoring board for a national clinical trial testing very large doses (megadoses) of antioxidant vitamins to see if they prevent cataracts and macular degeneration. Some physicians have remarkable faith in vitamins and believe that at least they can't hurt. They might urge their patients to take the large doses. Other physicians are professional skeptics. They would not want their patients to try the megadoses until there is evidence they are safe and effective. Still others may come down somewhere in between.

One physician's indifference point may be quite different from another's. The same patient whose physician is indifferent between a megadose of vitamins and a placebo could have seen another physician who firmly believes that the megadoses are the better option (or that the risks of harm make them more dangerous). The mere indifference of a patient's physician between two arms of a randomized trial does not after all seem to be adequate as a moral basis for justifying a randomization.

The Standard Answer, Part II: Indifference in the Clinical Community as a Whole

If the indifference of the individual clinician is not sufficient to provide a moral justification of a randomized clinical trial, perhaps we could make an adjustment. We could insist that in the clinical and scientific community[9] as a whole there is no clear preference for one treatment or another. The clinical community may be ambivalent or relatively indifferent about a treatment choice even if an individual clinician has a strong preference. More objective standards have generally replaced subjective clinician judgment as the basis for clinical decision making. If we replaced the subjective indifference of the individual clinician with an apparently more objective consensus within the scientific community as a whole that there was indifference between the two treatment arms, we might have a more legitimate basis for justifying the individual physician's recruitment of a patient into a randomized clinical trial.

When I was a young staff member at the Hastings Center in the early 1970s, I had a graduate student who interned with me who was interested in the ethics of clinical trials. He was particularly interested in the moral justification of randomization. His name was Benjamin Freedman. We spent many hours fighting over these issues, and his analysis was particularly provocative. He went on to publish in 1987 a famous paper in the *New England Journal of Medicine* based, in part, on the issues we discussed.[10] In it he introduced the concept of *clinical equipoise*. According to Freedman, what is critical is equipoise within the clinical community, not in the mind of the individual physician.

As he puts it, there must be "present or imminent controversy in the clinical community over the preferred treatment."[11] In order to keep this notion separate from the indifference of the individual physician, I shall here refer to Freedman's concept as *clinical community equipoise*. Because individual clinician opinion is not scientifically significant, Freedman says it is morally acceptable for a clinician to rely on the ambivalence within the community as a whole in proposing a randomized trial to her patients even if she personally prefers one of the treatment arms.

This was the standard wisdom circa 1987. A physician was morally justified in asking his patient to participate in a randomized clinical trial if the clinical community as a whole was legitimately ambivalent about the answer to the question of which treatment option was preferable, that is, if there was clinical community equipoise. This move to a community standard was seen as more objective than individual clinician judgment. It also permitted physicians to recruit patients for trials even if they themselves had an inclination one way or another that one of the treatments was preferred. It, of course, violated the Hippocratic Oath, because the physician was no longer working solely for the benefit of the patient, but it was a minor violation because one could honestly say that even though the research procedures were not undertaken for the patient's benefit, they were not significantly contrary to the patient's interest either.

The New Dilemma

This 1987 consensus, however, was not without its problems. Four issues are worth attention: *(1)* a lingering commitment to the full force of the Hippocratic Oath, *(2)* a dispute over the relation between scientists and clinicians, *(3)* a debate over the terminology of equipoise and indifference, and, most critically, *(4)* a controversy over why indifference or equipoise of the clinical community is morally relevant.

A LINGERING HIPPOCRATISM

Some clinicians remained so Hippocratic that they continued to feel guilty if they asked a patient of theirs to be randomized when they had a personal preference for one treatment over the other even though the clinical community was ambivalent. They failed to see that their idiosyncratic preferences for one treatment had little validity when their colleagues confronted with the same choices had no clear pattern of preference.

SCIENTIFIC VERSUS CLINICAL AMBIVALENCE

There was also lingering ambiguity in the concepts themselves. For example, at times Freedman writes as if the equipoise within the medical community had to be over some question of science.[12] According to this view, if medical scientists disagreed about which of two treatments would produce a greater rate of some outcome (such as survival), then the scientific community would in equipoise. This might be termed *scientific community equipoise*. At other times, however, he clearly is referring not to some dispute about a scientific question, but rather a disagreement about the value of two treatments. He defines *equipoise* as involving uncertainty about the "preferred treatment."[13] Here the disagreement is not over some question of science, but over the value of the outcomes. This is what I have called *clinical community equipoise*. Freedman attempts to make clear in later papers that he is interested in the latter as a basis for justifying randomization.[14]

Another young philosopher/bioethicist at Michigan State University named Fred Gifford took up these problems. He makes clear that scientific community equipoise and clinical community equipoise are two different matters. He also reaffirms Freedman's view that there is a difference between a community being exactly balanced between two options (what Freedman calls *theoretical equipoise*) and a lesser or "less fastidious" state in which there is no consensus within the expert clinical community, even though it may not be exactly balanced (what Freedman calls *clinical equipoise*).[15] Gifford presses the analysis further in a later paper, making clear that the theoretical/clinical distinction is not the same as the individual/community distinction.

DISPUTES OVER TERMINOLOGY:
INDIFFERENCE VERSUS EQUIPOISE

This disagreement spilled over into the terminology itself. Some have suggested that equipoise is best used to refer to the lack of consensus in a scientific community about some question of scientific fact whereas indifference was better reserved for the disagreements about value. If the medical community can agree about the outcomes of two treatments but remains ambivalent about which is the preferred package of benefits and harms, then the term *indifference* might be used.

There is something to this linguistic convention. I, however, prefer to speak more directly of uncertainty in the scientific community about a scientific question. I will reserve the term *indifference* to refer to ambivalence about the value of treatment outcomes. On the other hand, the term *ambivalence* can be applied in either situation.

My resistance to the term *equipoise* is not solely based on the confusion that exists because it might refer to either a scientific or a values dispute; it is also based on concern that the term is not one of ordinary language, especially outside the community of clinical trial experts. Speaking of *indifference* about which treatment's expected benefit/harm package is preferred I think is patently clear. One may be quite uncertain about some set of scientific facts and still very clear that one has a preference for one treatment option over another.

For example, if no one knew for certain whether quadruple bypass surgery produced better one-year survival than daily administration of aspirin for a certain group of patients, I take it that almost everyone would nevertheless under these circumstances have a clear preference about which treatment option they would choose. Precisely because no one is sure which produces a better outcome, patients would have a clear preference against the radical surgery. We could say in this situation that there was uncertainty about the scientific question and nevertheless physicians and their patients would not be indifferent about which of the two treatments they would choose. Given the dramatic difference in pain, suffering, inconvenience, and cost, the very fact that the scientific question was in dispute would lead many people rationally to prefer the aspirin regimen. They would not by any means be at their indifference points with regard to the two treatments.

Speaking of an *indifference point* better conveys that it is indifference that justifies randomization—that someone or some group must be more or less indifferent in evaluating the options for a randomization to be morally justified. At least they must see the difference as small enough that they are willing to risk forgoing the advantage of one of the treatments in order to contribute to science. Scientific uncertainty may be a necessary condition for a randomized trial to be justified, but it is not a sufficient condition.

I had been working with the concept of indifference since the 1970s when I was challenged in conversations with Charles Fried about these matters. I continue to prefer the term *indifference* over *equipoise*, at least when referring to ambivalence over which treatment option is preferred.

THE ROLE OF THE CLINICAL COMMUNITY

I was, however, never convinced that the indifference (or the equipoise) of the clinical community should be the proper moral basis for randomized trials any more than the ambivalence of the individual clinician should be. Here is where the problems with the old-fashioned modern medicine come to the surface.

In order to make a clinical judgment, two kinds of decisions must be made: judgments about the expected effects of each treatment and judgments about the value or disvalue of those effects. The latter are critical to the justification of a randomization, and they are, in principle, not judgments about which either scientists or clinicians are expert.

Judgments about the Effects of a Treatment

The first kind of judgment is by and large the province of medical scientists.[16] It is the role of clinicians to understand and convey the community consensus about the facts of medicine. The medical-scientific community should estimate likely effects of the treatment options, taking into account clinical anecdote, animal studies, past human trials, and theoretical models, as well as formal clinical trials.

If the consensus of the relevant scientific community is that a radical mastectomy is not known to produce a greater rate of survival from breast cancer than a lumpectomy, that seems, at least at first, to be the best estimate a society can use for justifying a randomization. We can say that there is uncertainty on the empirical scientific question. I say "at least at first." I will explain why below and take up the problem in more detail in chapter 22.

Judgments about the Value of Effects

In order to be indifferent between two proposed treatments, it is not enough to be legitimately uncertain about the facts, for example, over the question of which produces the higher survival rate. It may not even be necessary to be ambivalent. One must take into account other matters of medical fact: what the side effects are, for example. More critically, one must also take into account the evaluations of the outcomes. In the example of a radical mastectomy versus a lumpectomy, it should be obvious that even if the survival rates are the same, the two treatments are not equally attractive.

Some will defend radical mastectomy because they value the extra comfort from knowing that more of the potentially cancerous tissue was removed. Some on the other side will point to the obvious advantages of the lumpectomy: the psychological and cosmetic advantages, as well as more minimal trauma from the surgery.

In fact, if one believed there were no reason to hope for greater survival from a radical procedure, no one would consider it an option. For one to be indifferent between a radical procedure and a lumpectomy, one must consider the obvious advantages of the lumpectomy to be just offset by the hope for added survival from the radical procedure.

However, the trade-off between hope for added survival of the radical and the social/psychological attractiveness of the more modest procedure is a subtle, subjective one. Even among good scientists, there is no rational reason why people should have to agree on exactly which trade-off is the correct one. This is where postmodern medicine parts company with more traditional approaches. Postmodern medicine holds that physicians cannot be expert in deciding the value of the treatment alternatives even if they are expert on what is known about the likely outcomes.

In the scientific community one would expect some to prefer the radical and some the simple procedure. But here's the rub: On average, the members of the scientific community may not make these trade-offs the same way the members of the patient population might. There are more males among the scientists than among the patients who are candidates for mastectomy. There may well be more fear of death among them as well. There is no reason why this would not be reflected in the scientific community's indifference point. There is every reason to be concerned that if the patients assumed the scientists' understanding of the data, they could still not have the same indifference point as the clinical scientists.

Now let us return to the assumption that the clinical community should at least be considered authoritative in estimating the likely outcome from each of the treatments. Even if its members are not expert in placing values on the outcome, should they not at least be considered definitive in making the best estimate of the outcomes of the treatments in a clinical trial?

Granted, the clinical community does not know the outcome data definitively (or there would be no reason to conduct the trial), but it must at least determine its advance estimate of the outcomes, its prior probabilities, to use Bayesian language.

But there is a problem. People's prior probability estimates will be contingent upon their idiosyncratic beliefs and values. Particularly when estimates must be made based on admittedly inadequate data, personal, philosophical, and social beliefs will shape the way that scientists construct the problem, the data they rely on, and the way they describe the outcomes.

Thus, different members of the clinical community will estimate the facts about the outcomes differently, not just the value of the outcomes. And the way they estimate and describe those facts will be contingent upon their beliefs and values. Moreover, laypeople may hold beliefs and values that would have led them to different formulations of the estimates about the facts.

Even if we ignore the complex problems of the impossibility of a value-neutral account of the beliefs about the facts, the only reasonable conclusion is that patients and subjects can be expected to have indifference points that are different not only from individual clinicians but also from the clinical community as a whole. There is no reason why the patient or subject should be indifferent in choosing between two possible treatment options just because the clinical community is ambivalent. On the other hand, the patient or subject may be indifferent even when the clinical community has reached a consensus. In the next chapter, I try to work out of this conundrum.[17]

Drifting Out of Equipoise

Before proposing a way out of this dilemma, we need to address one last problem with the clinical community equipoise analysis. Fred Gifford, whom I mentioned earlier, addresses the fact that the clinical community will gradually drift out of equipoise between the treatment options so that it is no longer indifferent at some point before the end of a trial. This is a problem of randomized clinical trials that has long concerned me and others.[18] The goal of a trial is to produce statistically significant evidence that one treatment arm is superior to another. It is necessary to continue to accumulate data not just until one is nudged away from indifference between the options, but all the way until an adequate level of statistical significance is reached to be quite certain that there is a difference between the options. But before that point is reached, researchers and anyone else privy to the data will begin to realize there is a greater and greater probability that one arm of the trial is producing a preferable result. For example, in some trials, scientists use statistical tests to determine when a difference has been established adequately. They talk of "p-values" (the probability that the difference could have occurred by chance). The smaller the p-value, the less likelihood the difference was just random variation.

For some studies, a p-value of 0.05 is considered low enough to claim that one treatment is better than the other. But this creates a problem. Just before one reaches a p-value of 0.05, one will pass through p-values of 0.07 and 0.06. These can be interpreted as showing that there is a very substantial likelihood that the differences found are not occurring by chance. The difference would happen only seven or six times in a hundred if the treatments were really not different. Nevertheless, a good scientist wants to push on until some predetermined stopping criterion, such as a p-value equal to 0.05, is reached. Only at that point can one have an adequate level of confidence in one's conclusions to announce that a difference has been established with some certainty.

The clinician's task is radically different. He or she must facilitate a forced choice at a given moment for a particular patient. Often this must occur before the definitive data are available, but after one could conclude at some lesser level of significance that one treatment produces a better outcome than the other. This rationally provides a basis for preferring one treatment over the other (assuming one must choose before more definitive information is available).

The clinician and patient often must decide which of the two potential treatments looks more attractive before all the evidence is in. The clinician who is adequately informed will typically drift out of his or her zone of complete indifference regarding what is better for a particular patient before the randomized study can be completed. Because clinicians' primary loyalty must be to their patients, they are duty bound, if forced to make a choice, to choose the apparently more attractive arm. Although they cannot say they know for sure which is better, they are obliged to choose the apparently more attractive option. They are no longer indifferent.

In these situations, it truly is immoral for the physician to continue recruiting patients based on the grounds that either the individual physician or the clinical community is at their indifference points. They are no longer completely indifferent; they are not even approximately indifferent. Even if the matter is not completely decided, the balance has been tipped. If one were completely indifferent before the preliminary data were revealed—if the prior probabilities were equal—then any new evidence will upset that balance in one direction or the other. Although, as we have suggested above, very slight tilts in one direction may pose such a small preference that, with the patient's consent, randomization is still morally tolerable, there will often be cases in which clinicians have moved well beyond approximate indifference, although still not reaching the stopping boundary for the trial. There could be cases in which one drug appears to be saving a life whereas the other is not, and the difference could have occurred by chance only six times in a hundred. No rational person can be indifferent between these two drugs if a choice must be made at that point.

If the research moves at a slow enough pace that one can see interim data of this sort, it will never be possible to complete the research. It would be immoral to recruit patients into research on treatments that serve significant interests (like saving their lives or treating significant disease) if one treatment has a much greater likelihood of being better. Even though the apparently losing treatment still has a chance of proving equal or better, it is much more likely to end up the loser. Modern medicine has no way out of this dilemma. In the next chapter we will see that postmodern medicine has a solution.

| Randomized Human Experimentation

A Proposal for the New Medicine

Given the unexpectedly bleak turn in the recent history of the concept of indifference (or equipoise) as the justification for randomization, what should be done to salvage these crucially important trials? Both individual clinicians and the clinical community will typically drift out of equipoise long before an adequate level of certainty has been reached to conclude that we know one treatment is better than another. Reasonable patients will have a real interest in betting on the apparently winning treatment. Reasonable clinicians bound to promote their patients' interest will be obliged to tell them which treatment has the better odds. As long as benefit is conceived of as a matter of objective medical fact that can be known by competent clinicians informed by the latest research findings, no study of moment will ever be completed.

It will not do to adopt a strategy of keeping patients and their clinicians ignorant of the preliminary data trends because the core notion of informed consent for research requires that patient-subjects be told information that is potentially meaningful. If there was ever a piece of information that was potentially meaningful, it would be the knowledge that in preliminary analysis one life-saving treatment is doing better and the difference could have occurred by chance only six or seven times out of hundred. If the treatment serves important purposes for the patient—such as saving life or curing serious illness—no rational person would agree to being kept ignorant of this information.

The solution to this problem lies in the recognition that deciding which treatment best serves the patient's interest is not something a physician or group of physicians can know independent of the patient. Neither individual clinician indifference nor the indifference of the clinical community is sufficient to show that an individual patient with idiosyncratic interests should be indifferent. Patients who are not close enough to being indifferent that they agree to be randomized should not be made subjects of a randomized clinical trial even if their physicians or the clinical community as a whole really can't see an advantage to one of the treatment options. On the other hand, if it is possible for some group of patients to be honestly indifferent enough to the treatments that they consent to being randomized, the presence or absence of clinician indifference doesn't matter.

I propose that if the potential subject is willing to be randomized after being adequately informed and is not manipulated or exploited in the process, that is enough to provide a moral basis for randomizing. The new medicine provides a basis for understanding why it could be reasonable for some potential subjects to volunteer even if the clinical and scientific communities are no longer indifferent between the treatment options.

Differentiating Justifications for Research from Justifications for Randomization

First, I would urge differentiating the role of community uncertainty in justifying research from its role in justifying randomization. There are important moral questions about medical and other scientific research that have nothing to do with randomization. Budgets are limited. Not every research project that can be conjured up is worth pursuing. In fact, some would be immoral to pursue, not because they risk harm to subjects but because they squander scarce resources. Uncertainty in the scientific community plays a key role in deciding which research projects are worth pursuing.

We can start with the crude claim that for scientific research to be justified, there must be some scientific question that the research could answer. In order for there to be a question worth pursuing, there must be legitimate doubt about it. The distinction between scientific and clinical community equipoise is useful in helping decide whether there is a scientific question that is in doubt. As a first approximation, normally only if there is doubt in the scientific community is there a question that could be answered by the research.[1] That, of course, does not imply that if there is a scientific question that is open, it necessarily ought to be pursued. Some questions about which there is legitimate scientific doubt may nevertheless be quite irrelevant in the eyes of the community.

Determining whether the question is worth pursuing should bring the judgment of the lay community into the question. Only if the lay community, the ones whose resources will be consumed, considers the answers worth having should public or other community resources be invested. Even if the clinical or scientific community as a whole is in doubt about a question, it is still not worth pursuing if the lay population can envision no value in resolving the question.[2]

Justifying Randomization: The Role of Individual Subject Indifference

Thus the ambivalence, equipoise, or indifference of the scientific community is important in justifying the pursuit of a scientific question. The interest of the lay community is, as well, although for very different reasons. Neither of these, however, justifies randomizing a particular patient in a clinical trial. The individual who is a potential subject may have a strong preference between two treatments even if the broader lay and professional communities may see no basis for choosing between them. It is the individual subject who is randomized. It is he or she who runs the risk of ending up in an arm of the trial that may be, to him or her, unattractive.

A clinician is morally justified in entering a patient in a randomized clinical trial if, and only if, that individual patient after being adequately informed is approximately indifferent between the two treatment options or is otherwise willing to take the risk of receiving what to him or her is the less attractive option.[3] This is independent of individual physician's preference for one or the other of the treatments. It is independent of the clinical community's preference for one or the other. It is independent of the lay community's preferences.

What is critical is that the subject, after being adequately informed, does not have a clear preference for one or the other of the treatment arms or if she has a preference, she is willing to forgo that perceived advantage for the good of the·community. A potential subject may have a rational, if subjective, preference for one treatment arm or the other, even if the members of the clinical community have real doubt about the outcome and even have real indifference to which treatment they would prefer if they were the subjects of the study. One can, therefore, never assume that the individual subject will be indifferent just because the clinician or the community of clinicians is.

THE JUSTIFICATION

As I have argued throughout this book, one crucial finding in the evolution of medical ethics of the past 30 years is that physicians cannot know on their own which treatments will benefit patients and how much good various treatment options will do. This is not only, or even primarily, because they cannot predict perfectly what the outcome of various treatments will be: it is because the amount of good or harm a treatment does is fundamentally not a question of medical science. It is not something that is part of generalized clinical knowledge. The value of an outcome of a treatment is inherently a subjective matter based on the patient's idiosyncratic beliefs and values. The exact same outcome in two different patients may be valued by them quite differently. Hence, the old Hippocratic dictum that the physician should choose for the patient what will benefit the patient fails. The physician cannot know, in advance, whether a specified outcome will be valued by the patient or not. If a physician wants to know whether a treatment will benefit the patient, he will have to describe the anticipated effects and ask the patient.

The same is true for the treatment arms in a randomized clinical trial. A physician may have his or her own personal views about the values of anticipated outcomes. He or she may be indifferent between the two treatments based on the best estimate available of the expected outcomes. However, when physicians evaluate the expected risks and benefits of each arm in a clinical trial, they cannot know whether patients reach the same conclusions.

The physician's estimate of the benefits and harms is not definitive. The consensus of the clinician community is not definitive, either. Even the consensus of the lay community is not. It is the patient that counts. She may evaluate the outcomes differently. For those researchable hypotheses about which there is sufficient ambivalence in the scientific or clinical community to justify proposing a randomized clinical trial and there is sufficient interest in some lay community to warrant funding, giving the potential subject the opportunity to decide whether he or she is willing to participate is clearly justified. If, and only if, the subject is approximately indifferent (or willing to sacrifice for the good of science) can that subject justifiably be randomized.

An Adolescent with Leukemia

I once participated in the evaluation of a randomized trial designed to see if there was a difference between a three-year and a two-year drug regimen for adolescents with leukemia. The three-year regimen was the standard treatment. There were reasons to suspect, based on animal models and other sources, that administering the same regimen for two years would produce results that were just as good. If these suspicions were correct, the young patients could be spared a year's worth of the misery of the chemotherapy and the savings would be substantial. There was a risk that the two-year regimen would not be as effective, but, all things considered, the oncologists believed that the risks were small and justified by the potential benefits to the patients. The investigators were at their indifference points. Moreover, the community was persuaded that the investment was worth it. There seems no reason to doubt that they were justified in conducting the trial.

The problem arose in one 16-year-old patient. She and her mother were thoroughly informed of the risks and benefits as well as the design of the trial. After being given ample opportunity to ask questions, they were asked whether they were willing to have the girl randomized to receive either the two- or three-year regimen. The girl assented, and the mother gave her permission.

Because the effects of the drugs were powerful and unpleasant, there is no way this study could have been done on a double-blind basis. Both subjects and investigators knew from the start which arm the subject had been assigned.

When the results of the randomization were told to the girl and her mother, the girl was devastated to learn that she had been randomized to the three-year arm, in other words, the current standard of care. She burst into tears realizing that she would bear the nausea, vomiting, and all-important hair loss for an additional year.

The situation is an intriguing one. The investigators in all honesty believed that the benefits and harms of the two arms were evenly balanced. The girl clearly thought otherwise. Moreover, had she realized it, she had a clear right to the arm she preferred. She could drop out of the study, receive the standard treatment outside the protocol, and quit taking her three-year regimen after the second year. Alternatively, she could enter the trial and exercise her right to withdraw after the second year. Assuming she agreed to be followed by the study (asking that the subject continue to be followed is the standard practice when a subject exercises her right to withdraw), she would even continue to receive all the monitoring and other benefits of the study.

An ethics consultation focused on this newfound realization that the girl and her mother did not understand that due to the nature of the trial design, they had the right to get what the girl wanted. Equally interesting, however, is the demonstration that the honest indifference of the researchers and presumably of the rest of the scientific community did not imply that all the subjects in this study would also be at their personal indifference points. The adolescent, for her own reasons, found the hair loss and nausea sufficiently awful that they more than offset any marginal benefit of the possible extra chance of cure of the leukemia from taking the drugs for the third year. Her trade-off of this risk-benefit package was clearly different from that of the investigators. She was not truly at her indifference point when invited to enter the trial, even though the investigators, the clinical community, and the rest of society may have been at theirs.

At first, clinicians might be troubled by this suggestion that she could be permitted unilaterally to choose the treatment arm she preferred. They might believe it is irrational or even dangerous for her to pursue her preference when it had not been established that the two-year arm was as effective as the three-year arm. That conclusion, however, would be erroneous. From the point of view of the investigators, she loses nothing by insisting on what she prefers. The hypothesis of the study is that the two-year arm does not differ in effectiveness from the three-year arm. The investigators themselves accept the null hypothesis. They have to hold that they do not believe that the subjects getting the two-year arm are worse off than those getting the three-year arm. If they deny this, they are denying their null hypothesis and the study is immoral.

If the patient prefers one of the arms, in this case she should get it. She doesn't necessarily have the right to get it in the trial. I have elsewhere made the argument that it is actually better science to permit nonrandomized access to patients who prefer one of the treatment arms.[4] I will not pursue that here. Whether the subject gets access to the treatment inside the protocol or outside it, she should have the right of access to it. She is not at her indifference point and should not be randomized. In this case, all the patient has to do is start the three-year regimen and then stop after two years.

More generally, if patients, after being informed, have a subjective preference for the standard treatment, they should get it. They can do so by simply refusing to consent to being in the study. In that case, they will get the standard treatment. If they prefer the experimental treatment, they should get it on a nonrandomized basis within the protocol if that is feasible and, in most other cases, should get it through a compassionate use exemption, a treatment IND, an off-label use, or otherwise outside the protocol if that is possible. These are all mechanisms whereby patients with good reasons to get access to experimental drugs can obtain them.

Three Implications

The use of the individual subject's indifference point as a justification for randomization has three important implications for clinical trials: (*1*) It addresses the problem of discrimination against pro-innovation patients, (*2*) relying on individual subject indifference points as the justification for randomization provides a basis for solving the moral problem of completing trials, and (*3*) there is a possibility that we can manipulate personal indifference zones.

THE PROBLEM OF DISCRIMINATION
AGAINST PRO-INNOVATION PATIENTS

First, it addresses the problem of discrimination against pro-innovation patients. Right now we recognize that some conservative patients prefer not to enter trials even though the clinical community considers the experimental treatment equally attractive to the standard one. We give conservatives a right to opt out and get the standard treatment. This biases the sample somewhat, but we live with that consequence in the name of respecting patient autonomy.

If the experimental treatment is available outside the trial, we right now may also give patients a right of nonrandomized access. We presently do not give such pro-innovation patients a right of access to experimental agents that are not otherwise available to them, but if the agent is available over the counter, the patient has access. If it is available on prescription for other uses, the clinician has the right to prescribe for an off-label use and may be inclined to do so. Even if it is only available for research purposes, an investigator may see the wisdom of making the treatment available using a treatment IND or compassionate use exemption.

Often, however, patients who have a preference for the experimental agent cannot gain access. Hence, we discriminate against pro-innovation patients.

Even though the clinical consensus is that the new therapy has a risk/benefit profile that is equally attractive when compared with the standard therapy (i.e., the clinical community is at its collective indifference point), we often withhold access to the experimental treatment. Granting access to those who favor the experimental arm when supply is available eliminates discrimination and, I have suggested, produces better science. It eliminates the bias of permitting only those favoring the standard treatment to get access outside the protocol, and it permits scientists to examine whether the results of randomized access are similar to those from nonrandomized access.

THE PROBLEM OF COMPLETING TRIALS

Second, relying on individual subject indifference points as the justification for randomization provides a basis for solving the moral problem of completing trials. If we rely on clinical community indifference or equipoise as the justification for randomization, we have to acknowledge that typically the clinical community will cease to be indifferent between two treatment options before randomized trial has reached statistical significance. In these cases, it is immoral to complete the trial. Thus, most clinical trials today become immoral before they are completed. Only trials that begin and end so quickly that there is no chance for the reassessment of preferences escape this moral quandary.

I see only one solution to this problem: relying on individual subject indifference points to justify randomization. Individual patients are at their individual indifference points at different times during the evolution of a therapy. Many potential subjects, if informed, will share the evaluations of the clinical community and be at their personal indifference points at the inception of the trial. It is ethical to randomize them. (They would have no basis for choosing if they were not randomly assigned a treatment.) Some potential subjects, however, are not indifferent at the inception of the trial. They may find the anticipated side effects of one of the treatments unusually offensive or attractive. They may find an expected risk-benefit profile of one of the arms more attractive than most people do. Those who prefer the standard treatment have a right to get it. Those who prefer the experimental treatment normally should have a right to get what they prefer. They should not be randomized.

However, as the trial progresses, new information will become available from both inside and outside the trial. That new information should begin to push investigators and mainstream subjects out of their zones of indifference in the direction of one of the arms.[5] But as that happens, some people who formerly had a preference for the other arm may be nudged toward indifference. If the experimental arm begins to look attractive, some conservatives who originally preferred the standard treatment may begin to have doubts. If the experimental arm begins to look unattractive, some of those who earlier would have preferred it may rethink their preference. Both subjects and investigators will drift in and out of their personal indifference zones as the trial progresses. If the investigators can catch subjects as they drift through their personal indifference zones, it is ethically acceptable to randomize them *even if the investigators themselves have drifted out of indifference.*

As long as a scientific or clinical question has not been settled definitively, researchers ought to be able to find some subjects who are indifferent between the treatment options. The obligation of the investigators is to find those people and randomize them, while at the same time refraining from pressuring those who are no longer indifferent into consenting to enter the trial. What is morally relevant is individual patient willingness to be randomized and for any question of medical science that remains in significant dispute, there should be some group of patients who are legitimately indifferent. Find them, and they can be randomized even if it is immoral to randomize most other patients.

THE POSSIBILITY THAT WE CAN MANIPULATE
PERSONAL INDIFFERENCE ZONES

Suppose a researcher has too much trouble finding people as they drift into or out of their personal indifference zones. Can the researcher do anything to manipulate that indifference? This was the problem addressed by a graduate student at the Kennedy Institute of Ethics.

Julia Pedroni, now at Williams College in Williamstown, Massachusetts, has proposed in her doctoral dissertation that if not enough people can be located who are indifferent enough to be willing to be randomized, we should make offers to them to encourage them to be more indifferent.[6] She is not proposing that we lie to them about the risks and benefits of the treatment arms. Rather, she proposes that we offer incentives to them to make them more willing to be randomized. We might, for example, pay people to enter a trial, letting the market set the amount so that eventually the payment makes the consent to being randomized attractive enough. Or we might randomize people but pay them at the end of the trial if they get randomized to the losing arm (or the arm they had once found less attractive).

She points out that this is good, free-market economics. She also points out that our society does this all the time. If we need a worker during construction of a high-rise to walk around on the exposed beams on the twentieth floor, we enable them to find that work more attractive by increasing the pay in comparison to nice, safe ground-level construction. We make them more indifferent between the two jobs; in fact, we sometimes make the riskier job more attractive in comparison by piling enough money on the scales to tip the balance. Dr. Pedroni proposes that we manipulate indifference among potential randomized trial subjects in a similar way until we get enough volunteers to complete the trial.

This proposal is, of course, controversial. Some would say that such offers are coercive. However, current theories of coercion and respect for autonomy deny that attractive offers, even irresistibly attractive ones, are coercive.[7] Especially if all we do is drive a person into his or her personal zone of indifference (which is all we need to do to even slightly altruistic people), it is hard to claim we have coerced a person into volunteering to be randomized. In fact, we could claim that prior to providing the incentive, the person was lacking in real options because one of the treatment arms was so unattractive that the person had no choice.

I am not advocating that we adopt Julie Pedroni's free-market solution to the ethical problem of recruiting enough subjects to complete a clinical trial; however, she takes the subject of personal patient indifference points and develops a set of arguments that is harder to refute than it may appear.

I am personally inclined to hold to the norm that subjects should be compensated only for time and inconvenience. Usually the same amount of time and inconvenience is involved for all arms of a study. I prefer to recruit subjects for clinical trials by recognizing that the moral justification for their involvement must be that they are more naturally in their personal zones of indifference. Provided one recognizes that evaluation of risks and benefits of treatment options is inherently, inevitably subjective and that no clinician can ever determine when the patient ought to be indifferent without incorporating the patient's value preferences, we can see that different patients will drift in and out of their personal zones of indifference at different times.

Just when the clinician and his community drift out of indifference (and perhaps many of their patients drift along with them), some patients who previously had a rational, atypical preference for one of the arms will be forced into their personal indifference zones. The way to make randomized clinical trials ethical is by finding patients when they are at or close enough to their personal indifference points. Personal subjective indifference points provide the moral justification for randomization as well as the basis for completing clinical trials. They should replace personal physician, clinical community, and lay community equipoise as the basis for justifying randomization.

TWENTY TWO

Clinical Practice Guidelines and Why They Are Wrong

As long as benefits and harms were assumed to be objective and knowable by clinicians independent of individual patient values, people believed that competent clinicians drawing on competent medical science could determine how much good each medical treatment would produce for each patient. Of course, not all outcomes were guaranteed, but based on probabilities, clinicians thought they could predict the likely outcome for each patient and, based on this calculation, decide what was best for the patient.

Making such calculations would, naturally, be very complex, normally beyond the capacity of individual physicians standing at the bedside. However, this does not mean that such calculations could never be attempted. Groups of medical scientists at places like the National Institutes of Health could assemble all the relevant data and carefully calculate the outcomes of all the possible treatments for various carefully defined classes of patients. These data could then be used to write formal plans telling clinicians which treatments were, statistically, the best for each group of patients.

This enterprise has actually been attempted. The general project is called *technology assessment*. It involves several steps. First, the practitioners attempt to gather together all the best research about the possible outcomes from various treatment options. These efforts, called *outcomes research*, can then be used to develop treatment plans to produce what doctors have determined are the best outcomes. The result is a massive set of products called *practice guidelines* or *treatment protocols*. In this chapter I want to show why, in a post-modern society, this project is doomed to fail. If doctors cannot know what is best, they cannot write guidelines or protocols that tell how to do what is best for patients.

Technology assessment is a systematically ambiguous term. Its ambiguity causes serious problems for policy makers and clinicians. On the one hand, *assessment* sometimes refers to the scientific study of the potential *effect*s of a medical intervention. As such, technology assessment is often thought in the ideal to be scientific, objective, and value free. On the other hand, *assessment* sometimes refers to judgments about the benefits and harms anticipated from medical interventions and when they should be pursued. They attempt to tell when a treatment is "medically indicated," "appropriate," or a "treatment of choice." They attempt to tell how patients should be "managed."[1] In this manifestation, *technology assessment* always necessarily involves value judgments. Even in the ideal case, as we have seen in previous chapters, deciding that something is *beneficial* or *harmful*, deciding something is *indicated* or *ought* to be used in particular circumstances, always has to involve judgments about values that in principle cannot be determined by science alone.[2] Words like *beneficial, harmful, indicated,* and *ought* necessarily convey evaluations that go beyond the scope of what modern practitioners of science consider scientific.

Determining what the expected effect of an intervention will be can never, in principle, tell whether that effect is good or bad. It can never tell how the effect compares, in evaluative terms, with other options. Any assessment of technology assessment will have to provide an adequate understanding of the relation between knowing the effects of a treatment and knowing how valuable the treatment is. Without knowing the value of the treatment one can never, in principle, know whether the treatment is worth pursuing.

The Function of Technology Assessment: The Received Wisdom

The critical question is, "Is technology assessment supposed to provide facts without value judgment, or is it supposed to provide the necessary value framework for making medical decisions?" The received wisdom among many doing and using technology assessments is that high-quality, objective, scientific assessment of a technology will provide the basis for making correct clinical and public policy decisions. It is as if the generation of outcomes data, cost assessments, and other ideally objective findings based on impeccable scientific methodologies such as randomized clinical trials can lead directly to decisions about which treatments are appropriate in various medical circumstances.

Technology assessment is a general term covering a range of activities. Some, such as *outcomes research*, imply that the objective is to find facts, in particular to determine what the outcome will be from various interventions. If that were all there were to outcomes research, it would have the trappings of a scientific activity. It would provide data upon which clinicians, patients, and policy makers could impose a set of values to determine whether the expected outcome is worth pursuing. For example, the Patient Outcomes Research Team (PORT) studies, funded by the federal government's Agency for Health Care Policy and Research (AHCPR; now called the Agency for Healthcare Research and Quality), sought to establish the outcomes of treatment intervention such as whether radical prostatectomy and radiation therapy have an effect on localized prostate cancer.[3]

However, other techniques sometimes thought of under the rubric of technology assessment make clear their intention is to go well beyond fact finding. *Practice guidelines* or *treatment protocols* clearly imply that the goal of their creators is to direct a treatment course or at least guide it. For example, in the 1990s the AHCPR produced a series of 19 *Clinical Practice Guidelines*, all of which provide not only detailed recommendations for treatment, but also statements of the goals or values to be pursued in "managing" patients.

Still other techniques sit ambiguously between the goals of fact finding and prescription. *NIH Consensus Development Conferences* have as their stated purpose that they are to "evaluate publicly scientific information concerning biomedical technology and arrive at a Consensus Statement that . . . will serve as a contribution to scientific thinking about the technology under consideration."[4] In fact, if one examines the questions posed by the organizers of these conferences, it is clear that they sometimes want the conferees to reach a definitive consensus on questions of fact. For example, the consensus conference "Gallstones and Laparoscopic Cholecystectomy" asked the apparently scientific question, "What are the results of laparoscopic cholecystectomy compared with open cholecystectomy and other available treatments?"[5]

Other times they ask questions that require bold and blatant value judgments by the conferees. The same gallstone conference asked, "Which patients with gallstones should be treated with laparoscopic cholecystectomy?"[6] This a question that required judgments about risks to first- and third-trimester fetuses, patients with end-stage liver disease, as well as more usual value judgments about whether anesthesia and other risks are justified by the envisioned benefits compared with the risks.

The conference "Dental Sealants in the Prevention of Tooth Decay" asked apparently factual questions such as "How effective are sealants?" but also asked clearly normative questions such as "what should be the research priorities for sealants and their implementation?" Some of the questions combined both factual and evaluative questions such as "What are the clinical procedures involved in successful sealant application, and what training and education are required?"[7]

The claim that technology assessment necessarily involves evaluative judgments is most easily demonstrated in treatment guidelines and other devices that lead to treatment recommendations. A recommendation, by its very nature, is a statement that contains some normative prescription. I begin this unmasking of these formal schemes attempting to guide physicians by exposing the logical structure of clinical decisions. After that, I will examine treatment guidelines and protocols to tease out their hidden (or sometimes not so hidden) value judgments. We shall see that all such documents necessarily go beyond the science. They evaluate the science and use somebody's values to decide what *ought* to be done in the light of the data. Then in the next chapter I will show that even outcomes research—the efforts simply to find the medical facts—will necessarily incorporate evaluative judgments. I will argue that even those who eschew value judgments necessarily incorporate normative and conceptual commitments that shape the data and inevitably frame the decisions that clinicians, patients, and policy makers reach.

The Theoretical Structure of Clinical Decisions

Any clinical decision can be reduced to a formal syllogism of the following form:

If conditions A, B, C, D, and E exist, then one should do X.
Conditions A, B, C, D, and E exist.
Therefore, one should do X.

The second premise, the minor premise, will always contain fact claims. The placeholders, A, B, C, and so forth symbolize medical fact claims that come from diagnostic tests, pharmacological facts, and the findings reported in outcomes research. Some of these will also be fact claims from other areas including law, economics, sociology, and psychology.

For example, for a patient with pneumonia, the minor premise might include medical facts that lab tests are positive for pneumococcal bacillus, that penicillin has a high rate of overcoming pneumonia with minimal side effects, that the patient reports no history of anaphylactic reaction to penicillin, and so forth. It could also include facts from other disciplines such as law. The fact that penicillin is a legally available drug with FDA-approved labeling and so forth and the economic fact that resources are available to obtain penicillin are relevant legal and economic facts. The medical facts include those of the sort that might be established in outcomes research. Modern medical science treats the medical fact claims as potentially knowable by objective science. To varying degrees, the legal, economic, and other facts are also viewed as objectively knowable.

Even if one assumes that the conditions in the minor premise are knowable by objective medical science, clearly the major premise is not. The major premise of the clinical decision-making syllogism must always contain a normative judgment such as represented in "one ought to do X." If the conclusion contains a prescription—a recommendation or order for a drug, surgical procedure, or any other action—the major premise has to contain a value judgment. The ought judgment cannot come directly from the science. It must be imported from some system of beliefs and values. In clinical decisions, historically the beliefs and values have often been the clinician's. In the late stages of modern medicine (in the late twentieth century) sometimes the values were supposed to be those of the clinical community or the medical profession as a whole. In postmodern medical ethics with a commitment to patient autonomy, it is increasingly obvious that it is the patient's system of beliefs and values that ought to be incorporated into the major premise. It really doesn't make any difference what the values are of the patient's physician or of the medical profession as a whole. In public policy decisions, the values of the broader society might serve this function.

Practice Guidelines and Treatment Protocols

Practice guidelines, treatment protocols, and other technology assessment devices that purport to guide, direct, recommend, or instruct clinicians in making decisions necessarily provide all three elements of the clinical syllogism. They draw on outcomes research, consensus conferences, and more traditional clinical trials to provide the medical data that fit into the minor premise.

It is the nature of practice guidelines and treatment protocols that they go beyond the medical facts supplied by the scientific disciplines related to medical research. First, although the writers of the guidelines and protocols often do not realize it, they incorporate purported facts from other disciplines. Consider, for example, whether protocols for metastatic cancer should include among the treatment options the possibility of physician-assisted suicide or euthanasia. Almost no protocols include that option, in part because it is correctly believed that such options are illegal or at least so immoral that they are not worth mentioning. Likewise, heroin is not a treatment option for severe pain, not because it is necessarily ineffective, but because it is correctly understood that heroin use is illegal in the United States. Sociological and psychological facts are also often incorporated into treatment protocols. They are among the conditions incorporated by implication in the minor premise.

Even if the writers of the protocols and the clinicians who use them can claim real expertise on the medical facts, they normally have no such claims to expertise on facts in other disciplines. Thus there is already some reason to be suspicious that groups that write protocols necessarily have the scientific skills necessary to support all the relevant facts for a clinical recommendation.

The more obvious implication of the clinical treatment syllogism is that even if the protocol and practice guidelines writers can assume that they have all the relevant facts of the minor premise correctly assessed in a value-free and reliable manner, they can surely make no such assumption about the major premise. It is the major premise that must provide a normative framework for all clinical decisions.

CASE 22.1

Penicillin for Pneumonia

The patient has a bacillary form of pneumonia and has no history of anaphylaxis. Should he take penicillin? True, almost all people reach that conclusion, but if they do, it is because they share a set of values that appraises the potential benefits and risks of the penicillin, compare those to the benefits and harms of other treatment options, and conclude that the effects of the penicillin are, on balance, better. That is not a scientific conclusion. It assesses the medical and other facts and imposes a set of external values on them to reach the conclusion that one ought to take the penicillin.

The nonscientific, normative nature of these decisions becomes apparent if one considers that a Christian Scientist might fully accept all the relevant facts of the minor premise and still deny that one ought to take penicillin. What is more important, some patients who make no special religious metaphysical assumptions may, under special circumstances, deny the moral and other normative content of the major premise.

A 90-year-old patient terminally ill with metastatic cancer may question whether it is better to take penicillin and live than refuse it and die. Medical science alone can never establish definitively that it is right to take penicillin when one has pneumonia.

If that is true for as simple a medical circumstance as pneumonia, it is more dramatically true when the values underlying the treatment options do not lead as obviously to a particular ought statement. Each patient brings unique values to a treatment decision. These unique values cannot be reflected in clinical practice guidelines.[8]

All practice guidelines and treatment protocols that recommend how a patient should be treated supply not only the diagnostic, prognostic, and pharmacological facts, but also the other relevant nonmedical facts as well as the religious, philosophical, or other normative values that lead to the judgments about how the patient should be treated.

For example, the guideline "Management of Cataract in Adults" includes the statement that the goal is to "maintain and restore autonomy through appropriate treatment to remove the disability."[9] This sounds reasonable to most of us, but it is not a fact; it is a value judgment. In the guideline "Management of Cancer Pain: Adults," the writers make the recommendation that "The clinician's ethical duty—to benefit the patient by relieving pain—supports increasing doses [of opioids], even at the risk of side effects."[10] Surely that is not a conclusion of medical science, no matter how plausible the ethical opinion is among many cultural groups.

In some of the guidelines, some evaluative judgments are more subtle but nevertheless clearly convey value choices. In the guideline "Depression in Primary Care: Detection, Diagnosis, and Treatment," the authors transfer some of the value choices to the clinician as when they say that "if panic disorder and major depression are both present and the panic disorder has been present without episodes of major depression in the past, the clinician must judge which is the most significant condition. . . ."[11] Why it is the clinician rather than the patient who must judge is not at all clear.

In the guideline "Managing Otitis Media with Effusion in Young Children," one of the many ways in which the value judgment of the writers is manifest is in how they handle the problem of whether to recommend intervention when the evidence of effect is not definitive. In discussing adenoidectomy for uncomplicated middle ear effusion in the child younger than age 4, when adenoid pathology is not present, they say that, "based on the lack of scientific evidence," the treatment is not appropriate.[12] However, on the previous page, when faced with a situation where they lack evidence, they reach the opposite conclusion, saying, "Although there is insufficient evidence to prove that there are long-term deleterious effects of otitis media with effusion, concern about the possibility of such effects led the panel to recommend surgery [bilateral myringotomy with tube insertion for the child who has had bilateral effusion for a total of 3 months and other conditions]."[13]

These are just a few of the countless evaluative judgments made in the practice guidelines. Every time a procedure is recommended, a value judgment is made that takes the authors beyond the science. It is not that the judgments are implausible; it is simply that they do not come from the data. The only plausible conclusion is that all attempts to formulate practice guidelines or treatment protocols necessarily import moral and other value judgments from religious, philosophical, and other systems of belief and value from outside medical science.

This helps explain why some clinicians offer resistance to treatment protocols, even those formulated by the Agency for Health Care Policy and Research and other bodies capable of providing the highest quality research in medical science. Although undoubtedly many clinicians deviate from the recommendations of protocols and guidelines because they hold beliefs about the medical data that do not conform to the data provided by the most reliable sources, even if they accepted the data and had perfect knowledge of it, they might still reject the values the writers used to make their recommendations. If one placed less value on autonomy of the elderly and more value on efficiency of those in the labor force, one might reach different conclusions about cataracts. If one had a strong commitment to preserving life, regardless of the pain, one might be less willing to risk side effects of opioids. It is not clear why the clinician's determination of whether panic disorder or depression is more "significant" should be the definitive value. It is also unclear why the panel's willingness to intervene in the face of insufficient evidence in one case but not the other should be definitive. Even if one knows exactly the effect of an intervention, one cannot directly conclude whether that effect is a good or a bad one or how the various value trade-offs should be made.

In the case of otitis media, the guideline makes clear that there is a statistically significant improvement in clearance of effusion (release of fluids from the infection) at one month, whereas there is no difference at two months and no evidence of prevention of long-term hearing loss. Physicians and parents facing a child screaming in pain form otitis media may place more emphasis on short-term effects than do researchers who can show that there are no measurable long-term effects from the infection. Even if the researchers have a perfect account of the effects of administration of an antibiotic, they must evaluate those effects. If the protocol writers focus exclusively on long-term effects while the clinician and parents also worry about the short-term, reversible consequences as well, both the clinician and the parents may rationally disagree with the writers of the protocol without denying that the writers have the best available estimate of the medical facts.

Just as clinicians may bring different values to the data than the protocol writers, so patients and their families may evaluate the outcomes differently from their clinician. That is why no clinician can ever know what is the best treatment for a patient without finding out what value system should be used for deciding benefits and harms. If we assume that the patient's values should be dominant in clinical decisions, then, as I have argued throughout this book, the only way that the clinician can know what is the best treatment for the patient is to ask the patient, that is, to ask the patient to evaluate treatment options and pick the one that fits the patient's value system.[14]

In the case of an incompetent patient who has never chosen and expressed a set of values, for pediatric patients with otitis media, for example, the choice of the proper value system is even more complicated. It is the parent or other familial surrogate who should be selecting the values, provided they are within reason.[15] It is normally up to public agencies—courts and child-protection agencies—to determine whether the family members must be overridden because they are beyond reason in judging what is in the incompetent patient's interest. In any case, there is no reason to assume that the clinician's values are the appropriate ones to impose on the medical data.

Thus, neither the protocol writers nor clinicians can be the definitive treatment decision makers. Even if we assume that the treatment protocol writing group has definitive expertise in deciding the relevant medical facts, it cannot be presumed to be authoritative in deciding which values to use.[16] In the next chapter I press the issue of whether values also have to play a role in establishing what the medical facts are.

TWENTY THREE

Outcomes Research and How Values Sneak into Finding of Fact

Even if clinicians and patients may rationally reject recommendations in practice guidelines and treatment protocols because they reject values incorporated into them, still many seem to believe that clinicians and patients ought to accept at least the fact finding in technology assessments. As we saw in the last chapter, many technology assessments are not so ambitious as to strive to make treatment recommendations. They claim only to be finding and reporting the relevant medical facts. If they could do that job, then the facts found in outcomes research could provide the data for the medical portion of the minor premise in the treatment syllogism. Outcomes research could provide the medical facts on which patients, clinicians, and public policy makers could impose their externally derived evaluations.

The logical function of outcomes research is to provide a consensus of expert medical researchers on the relevant medical facts about a particular medical intervention. This more modest function of technology assessment will admittedly not provide the leverage of more ambitious practice guidelines. It will not provide any basis for evaluating the facts and, logically, cannot provide any recommendations for treatment interventions. It cannot even supply all the relevant facts; it cannot supply the nonmedical facts necessary in any sound treatment decision. But outcomes research could, according to this more modest view of technology assessment, at least give us a scientifically sound basis for estimating the medical facts.

NIH-Sponsored Outcomes Research

In the 1990s the NIH agencies began sponsoring studies that seemed designed to measure outcomes. The Patient Outcomes Research Teams (PORT) and the consensus conferences are two examples.

PORT STUDIES

Agency for Health Care Policy and Research (AHCPR) sponsored a program to create patient outcomes research teams," to conduct research on the outcomes for various clinical interventions. Called PORT studies, they were conducted in two rounds (referred to as PORT-I and PORT II) and designed to focus primarily on outcomes. The announcement of the second round of PORT studies specified that the projects were to examine the effectiveness or cost-effectiveness for the prevention, diagnosis, treatment, and management of common clinical conditions.[1] They sought to compare two or more distinctly different clinical approaches, asking what the outcomes will be, not necessarily going on to ask which outcomes were worth pursuing.

Examples from the first round of PORT studies made clear that fact finding was a major objective. For example, the ischemic heart disease PORT found that something called the Duke Treadmill Score can identify between one-third and two-thirds of outpatients with chest pain who are at low risk for coronary artery disease. It also found that lower incidence of heart disease was the reason that women are not referred for cardiac catheterization as often as men rather than because of referral bias against women.[2] These both purport to be factual findings.

Interspersed with these factual findings, however, are treatment recommendations resembling the practice guidelines already discussed in the previous chapter. One report concluded that the benefits of thrombolytic therapy outweigh the risks of intracranial hemorrhage for most AMI patients and the U.S. physicians are unnecessarily reluctant to use thrombolytic therapy.[3] These surely are value judgments imposed on the data requiring comparison of the harms of heart attacks and stroke as well as value judgments about the relative importance of iatrogenic and naturally occurring medical problems.

Similarly, the prostate PORT strayed into occasional clinical recommendations. One published study concluded that watchful waiting is a reasonable alternative to invasive treatment for men 60 to 75 with localized prostate cancer, a judgment that requires assessment of the psychological anxiety of the wait as well as the alternative costs, something that cannot be gleaned from the scientific study.[4]

CONSENSUS DEVELOPMENT CONFERENCES

At least at first other efforts at the National Institutes of Health look like they are just pursuing questions of medical fact. The series of consensus conferences organized by the Office of Medical Applications of Research (OMAR) at the National Institutes of Health and other cosponsors is sometimes presented as striving to develop agreement on the medical facts of certain controversial medical technologies.[5] They differ from AHCPR outcomes research in that they do not involve their own empirical research on the technologies involved. A panel of leading experts with relevant technical expertise is assembled to hear empirical researchers present the results of their research. A series of questions is presented to the panel that, after listening to two to three days of testimony from leading researchers, goes into closed session to prepare a consensus on their perception of the relevant facts.

In spite of their charge, many of these panels do not restrict themselves to purely factual matters. Many consensus panels drift into clinical and public policy recommendations. In fact, many of the questions force them to do so. One would think that the more experienced organizers at OMAR and other agencies associated would understand the difference between apparently scientific questions on the one hand and clinical and policy judgments on the other, but often that is not the case.

The series of conferences has covered many major areas of medical technology. Usually the questions put to the panel include a number of important matters that would be perceived by most as questions of fact. The critical care medicine conference, for example, asked, "Is there empirical evidence that intensive care units cause a decrease in patient morbidity and mortality?"[6] The electroconvulsive therapy conference asked, "What is the evidence that ECT is effective for patients with specific mental disorders?"[7] The blood cholesterol panel asked, "Will reduction of blood cholesterol levels help prevent coronary heart disease?"[8]

But each of the panels is also asked some normative questions that require going far beyond the data: What critical care interventions should be routinely available? What factors should the physician consider in determining whether electroconvulsive shock is appropriate? Under what circumstances should dietary or drug treatment be started to treat blood cholesterol?

Value Judgments in Fact Finding

The NIH consensus development conferences have to be seen as a technology assessment method that incorporates some more direct explicit evaluations of the sort seen in practice guidelines and treatment protocols along with some questions that appear, at least to the naive observer, to involve questions of scientific medical fact. When pursuing these apparent questions of fact, these conference panels look like outcomes research projects. Many working with the model of modern medicine will assume that the consensus conference panelists, at least when they pursue their more restricted fact-finding function, can strive to be objective and value-free providers of medical facts, leaving it to others—clinicians, patients, or policy makers—to insert the evaluations.

Unfortunately, recent developments in philosophy of science and philosophy of medicine suggest that even this more modest function for technology assessment may face problems in being value free. The division of clinical reasoning into major and minor premises relies on what philosophers call the fact/value distinction. Its origins go back at least as far as David Hume. According to it, facts and values are conceptually distinct so that it is logically impossible to derive a value from a set of facts. In our case, it is logically impossible to derive the value judgment that a treatment ought to be used from the facts that, if it is used, a certain result is likely to be obtained. The "ought" necessarily comes from a different source than the "is." "Oughts" are imposed on the data from the outside.

But recent thought in philosophy of science is beginning to question this sharp separation. It is now widely believed that the doing of science itself necessarily incorporates conceptual and normative judgments that make all scientific propositions dependent on these judgments. Holders of this view claim that all statements that are presented as facts actually would be crafted differently if those articulating the statements had different conceptual and normative commitments.

There was a time when the belief prevailed that science at its best was, at least theoretically, objective and value free. Observations of facts were the source of knowledge about the external world that provided the foundation for confirming or refuting scientific hypotheses. The work of contemporary philosophers of science such as Ludwig Fleck,[9] Thomas Kuhn,[10] and Paul Feyerabend,[11] and fellow travelers in sociology of knowledge such as Thomas Luckmann and Peter Berger[12] and the postmodern critics of Hippocratic medical ethics[13] hold that theory construction in science and the doing of science are inherently dependent on a system of beliefs and values, a thought collective (Fleck), a paradigm (Kuhn), or a worldview.

The "paradigm" provides the conceptual system that articulates the metaphysical beliefs about the nature of reality, frames the questions being asked, determines which researchable questions are worth pursuing, provides the criteria for observation, establishes the methods of doing research, selects criteria for end points of research, identifies the way findings are reported, and provides the language by which science is communicated.

Just as the Ptolemaic and Copernican worldviews are incommensurable or the medieval world of faith sees reality differently from the modern world of reason, so the doing of science can be divided into two different enterprises. As Thomas Kuhn originally suggested in his now-famous *Structure of Scientific Revolutions*,[14] two periods occur in the doing of science: (1) There are moments of revolutionary science in which one paradigm begins to come apart and is replaced by another, and (2) there are periods of normal science in which the basic presuppositions are not questioned and puzzles are solved. When one paradigm replaces another, it is not possible to say that there has been progress. There are different worlds.

One of the most significant theses of post-Kuhnian philosophy of science is that accounts of the world offered by those in different worlds are incommensurable. Even the same words have different meanings. Recently adjustments have led to a distinction between (1) radical incommensurability and (2) local (or partial) incommensurability. Also efforts are under way to apply the notion of incommensurability to smaller, more local divisions in worldview so, for example, feminist medical scientists and Orthodox Jewish medical scientists can be said to see the world differently and both see something different than do more mainstream secular scientists. They ask different questions, have different criteria for proof, use concepts differently, and select different observations as worth recording and publishing.

These developments have important implications for outcomes research and other work in medical science. According to these theorists, medical scientists will necessarily incorporate their system of beliefs and values into the way they do their scientific research. Any account of reality will be framed by the underlying worldview and value system of the one doing the work. Other scientists with other worldviews would have shaped the problem differently, conducted investigations differently, ended up with a different account of the reality they are observing—not necessarily any better or worse accounts, just different. Their accounts will be incommensurable with an account of an apparently similar phenomenon seen from a different paradigm.

Anyone doing outcomes research will carry with that research a view of the world that will shape the account. Equally competent scientists with another worldview would have given a different account. It is like an artist and an auto mechanic each asked to give a brief description of a Maserati. The artist will describe the brilliant red color, the sweeping, graceful lines, and the streamlined proportions. The auto mechanic will tell us about the cubic centimeters of the engine, the torque, and the turning ratio. It is not that either is wrong; they are just different. Outcomes research will not be able to give a single, definitive description of what the effects of a medical intervention will be. Each scientist will have his or her story to tell, but they will be different stories depending on what each considers important.

Imagine a group of medical scientists gathered together in an NIH consensus conference for the purpose of generating a consensus on what the outcome will be of a group of medical interventions. The issue may be the outcome of lumpectomy versus radical surgery for certain specified breast cancers, whether dental sealants will reduce dental caries in children and by how much, whether nurse-midwife home birth is as safe as in-hospital deliveries under the supervision of an obstetrician. The panel members will not all come up with exactly the same assessments of these apparently factual matters. There will be a distribution of views.

Empirical research supports the claim that scientists with different values will give different accounts of the facts. They will be correlated with the scientist's beliefs and values. These are not to be attributed solely to bias or distortion. They are an inevitable result of the necessary influence of paradigm or world view on the doing of science. Moreover, there is no a priori reason to assume that any one estimate, say, the mean estimate, of the facts is the most likely to be correct.

Clinicians dealing with patients need an account of the medical facts to launch a consultation with the patient about alternative approaches to any medical problem. They will draw from the outcomes research in programs such as the PORT studies and consensus development conferences to provide what they take to be the most reliable, scientifically valid accounts of those medical facts. In spite of their best efforts to be fair and accurate, however, they will have to incorporate their beliefs and values in selecting from the huge amount of data the "important" or "worthwhile" information. They will have to simplify it, reducing it to a manageable account that patients can understand.

The first major project I undertook in the study of medical ethics was a study of physician communication to patients about birth control.[15] I was interested in how clinicians integrated their understanding of the relevant medical facts and their personally held values in order to make clinical recommendations to patients.

Doctor, Does the Pill Cause Cancer?

In the late 1960s the birth control pill was changing the lives of people throughout the world. Birth control was a controversial moral issue. It challenged the thinking of Catholics who held that only "natural" limits to fertility were acceptable. It challenged the deeply held beliefs of Protestants who believed that sexual relations should be limited to those within a marriage. It challenged the cultural commitment of Jews who believed they had a religious duty to "be fruitful and multiply."

I interviewed internists and obstetricians who had regular opportunities to counsel women about the momentous decision to begin using a new drug called the oral contraceptive. I also sent questionnaires to a group of their patients in order to determine their moral inclinations about birth control.

I asked the doctors questions that would be understood as questions of medical science, questions such as "How likely is a woman to become pregnant if she misses one pill during the middle of her cycle when she is most fertile?" and "Does the pill cause cancer?" These were hot questions of the day, and the answers were critical to determining whether women would choose to use oral contraceptives. I also asked the doctors questions about whether they thought birth control was morally acceptable, questions addressing the belief that fertility limits should be "natural," that oral contraceptives might increase promiscuity, and whether the pill was generally morally consistent with their religious values. Finally, I asked them questions about their general medical practices on such issues as whether they would initiate conversations about birth control with women in premarital exams or postpartum medical interactions.

My major finding was quite predictable: These practices, such as initiating conversations with patients about birth control, were more likely to occur if the doctor thought the pill was moral. The more provocative finding was that not only were the doctor's practices correlated with their moral views, their views about the medical facts were as well. If birth control pill was immoral, pregnancy was more likely to result from missing a pill. If it was immoral, it was more likely to cause cancer. Presumably, these "medical facts" were communicated to the patients. Anti–birth control doctors in interviews said, in effect, "I won't preach to you about the morality of the pill, but I can tell you that it can cause cancer." On the other hand, more liberal doctors would insist that there was no proof that the pill caused cancer.

One might be inclined to think that these differences occurred because physicians were letting their personal moral views bias their reading of the objective scientific evidence, that they were letting their ethics distort the existing medical literature. There is an inclination to ask what the "really true" facts are.

In fact, in interviews with the physicians it became clear that there was little, if any, evidence of misrepresentation of the scientific literature. The problem was more complex. Physicians, like all scientists, must select from a huge, unmanageable set of data and simplify it into a coherent, understandable story. In doing so, they naturally select what they take to be important information. It is that selection that requires a set of beliefs and values.

Conservative doctors could point accurately to data showing there were precarcinogenic cell changes in the breasts of beagles that were given the hormones in birth control pills. To them, this was "significant" information that women should take into account in deciding about oral contraceptives. Meanwhile, liberal physicians could state accurately that, at the time, there was no evidence that the pill had ever caused cancer in a human being. To them, that was the important information.

A more reflective critic might be inclined to say that the fair thing for a doctor to do would be to tell the patient both facts about cancer. The trouble with that, however, is that there not just two facts, there are potentially an infinite number of them. Some of them are so trivial that no reasonable person would want to hear about them. Some seem irrelevant; others seem marginal. Any clinician, or any scientist informing clinicians, must select from an infinite set of possible data, the "important" information, but what is important is necessarily determined by one's beliefs and values. Superimposing of a value framework on the facts is inevitable. Patients will get dramatically different accounts of the relevant medical facts depending on the values of the clinicians and scientists that are providing them.

One might be inclined to hope that this problem of values shaping the account of the facts was a problem limited to clinicians who have to communicate with laypeople who cannot manage large quantities of cutting-edge scientific data. This raises the question of whether frontline scientists and government science panels are similarly at risk for such shaping of scientific accounts. Do those high-level scientists involved in the PORT studies, consensus development panels, and similar strategies for articulating accounts of the medical facts avoid letting their personal values shape their accounts? Does the creation of a panel or group of scientists neutralize any distortions that might occur? That is the issue to be faced in the final chapter of this book.

TWENTY FOUR

The Consensus of Medical Experts and Why It Is Wrong So Often

Over the past two decades consensus formation among experts in the medical enterprise has had a controversial history. In the earliest, most naive stage, the belief was virtually universal that experts in clinical medicine could, by consensus, determine what were the correct clinical interventions for various conditions. Although this may still be the belief today among many ordinary clinicians as well as among patients and other laypeople, it is generally recognized by most who think critically about philosophy of medicine to contain logical errors. Earlier chapters in this book have shown why even the most expert clinicians in the world cannot, on their own, establish what is the proper clinical treatment for a particular patient.

Even among those who have long since realized that the consensus of experts in medical science cannot determine what is the clinically correct course for any given patient, there remains a willingness to turn to the consensus of experts in certain more policy-oriented tasks and more apparently scientifically oriented questions. In particular, "blue ribbon" panels of scientific or medical experts are often relied upon to perform two critical public tasks: First, panels are used to reach a consensus on certain evaluative tasks such as determining how funds should be allocated, whether drugs are safe enough to be on the market (with or without prescription), or whether professional behavior is within acceptable limits. Second, they are asked to reach a consensus on apparently technical factual questions.

This chapter argues that the same analysis that supports the conclusion that it is a mistake to attribute expertise to medical experts in making clinical decisions also forces the conclusion that groups of experts cannot justifiably be relied upon to formulate public policies related to their field of expertise or even to reach a reliable consensus on matters of fact within their area. Applied to medicine, the thesis is that it is a logical mistake to rely on experts in medicine to formulate public policies related to medicine or even to articulate the medical facts in their area of expertise.

Consensus of Experts in Public Bodies

At first it might seem reasonable to rely on the consensus of a group of medical experts in the public decision-making arena. Various public questions simply must be answered: How much and what kinds of information should a clinician tell a patient about the risks of a procedure to avoid being guilty in a court of law of treating without adequate consent?[1] Should more public money be spent on research on critical care medicine?[2] Is there empirical evidence for an effect of special diets on hyperactivity in children?[3] With what groups of patients should mood-altering drugs be considered for preventive maintenance medication?[4] Are dental sealants effective in preventing cavities in children?[5] Under what circumstances should coronary artery bypass surgery be considered?[6] These, in fact, are all questions that groups of experts have been asked to answer in various public bodies.

Groups of medical experts convene as advisory bodies to medical insurers (public and private), Congress, and executive branch agencies of government. One of the most important projects in consensus formation in medicine has been the long and important series of consensus conferences sponsored by the National Institutes of Health.[7] It has been widely assumed that if substantial agreement can be reached among a broadly constituted group of experts in a field about some question that seems clearly related to that field, then that consensus should have substantial significance. It should be viewed as a particularly reliable approximation of the truth with regard to the question being asked.

I challenge that assumption. It is at least critical to analyze further how the specific questions being asked relate to the real expertise of the members of the supposedly expert panel. Even in cases in which it seems most plausible that the presumption of expert knowledge is valid—that is, in the area of technical, scientific facts—there are theoretical reasons why panels of experts can be expected to reach the wrong conclusions. In order to make this case, I need to go back to the earlier debate over the involvement of medical experts in clinical judgments and the extent to which they can be presumed to have expertise in such judgments.

Clinical Generalization of Expertise: the Origins of Our Doubt

Among those more naive about the role of the consensus of experts in medicine, the first doubts about attributing to medical experts a knowledge in medicine arose in certain clinical cases involving what were clearly judgments of ethical significance. Beginning about 1970, many people became concerned that clinicians were presumed to have the ability to know what was the correct clinical decision for patients even in cases in which the significant issue seemed to be not so much medical science as moral evaluation of alternative interventions. The central theme of this book has been that relying on medical experts for these decisions has been a mistake.

Perhaps the most conspicuous case was that of aggressive life-prolonging treatment of terminally ill cancer patients whose lives could be extended somewhat with high-tech, burdensome treatments, but whose diseases could not be cured. Until about 1970, clinicians presumed to be the appropriate decision makers in such cases, and patients naively tolerated that presumption. At about that time serious doubt began to emerge about the presumption that expertise in the medical science of cancer automatically gave one expertise in the evaluative judgments about what ought to be done for cancer patients whose diseases could not be cured. Likewise, similar cases involving other chronic, incurable conditions forced the same question on us. Patients in an incurable persistent vegetative state like Karen Quinlan raised the question of whether it was worth it to prolong unconscious life,[8] and people began to doubt that experts in the neuroscience of persistent vegetative state (PVS) should be given authority to make the moral judgments about whether such life should be preserved.

Other clearly medical situations seemed to call for analogous judgments involving matters unrelated to science. Women were beginning to decide whether pregnancies should be maintained or prevented. People began asking whether kidneys should be transplanted and whether some genetic diseases were so horrendous that they justified ending the lives of their victims. Observers of clinical decision making gradually became convinced that being an expert in the medical science of these conditions did not give one the evaluative expertise to know what to do when they existed. Many years ago I gave the name *generalization of expertise* to the phenomenon of presuming that because one was an expert in the science of a particular condition, one was also an expert in the clinical evaluative judgments about what ought to be done about that condition.[9]

I shall assume that the reader of this book is by now convinced that it is an error to presume that expertise can be generalized in this fashion. Although it is possible that those who have scientific expertise in an area also possess wisdom in the evaluation on what ought to be done in that area, it is wrong to presume that such a link automatically occurs, that by the very process of becoming a technical expert in an area, one also acquires some special skill in making ethical and other value judgments about what one ought to do in that area. In fact, one might be so skeptical as to doubt that there is any such thing as evaluative expertise in medicine (or in any other area). I am not holding out for such skepticism here. I am claiming only that it is wrong to presume that technical expertise automatically gives one ethical and evaluative expertise.

To be sure, many to this day do not recognize this error. They especially do not recognize the error of generalizing the clinician's expertise in more routine, everyday medical decisions, those not involving more obvious, high-profile, ethical issues. They fail to see that when clinicians prescribe cough medicine or hernia surgery or penicillin for pneumonia, they are engaging in evaluative judgments that are logically independent of the scientific medical knowledge the clinician possesses. Nevertheless, I hope I have persuaded the reader that the naive acceptance of clinical generalization of expertise cannot be sustained even for these routine, apparently nonmoral value judgments. Eventually clinicians and laypeople will be persuaded that there is no logical link between medical training and the presumption of expertise in the value judgments needed to decide what ought to be done in any clinical situation. Even if physicians, as part of their training, learn a unique constellation of values that support clinical judgments, there is no reason to presume that these values are more correct or more appropriate, especially for patients who do not share them. The rejection of this presumption of generalization of expertise is the starting point of this "second generation" examination of expertise in medical decision making.

The Consensus of Expertise

If it is wrong to presume that a clinician is an expert in the value judgments necessary for clinical decisions just because he or she is an expert in the medical science of the patient's condition, it is a short step to the evolution of doubt about the significance of a consensus of a group of clinicians about what ought to be done about a particular class of patients. Getting one's colleagues together to develop a clinical consensus may help eliminate the idiosyncratic evaluations of a single clinician who may have a unique or distorted perspective. However, it cannot provide a sound basis for establishing the correct or appropriate evaluation of what ought to be done about a condition. For example, it does not follow from the fact that at one point in our recent history the vast majority of clinicians believed that painful, metastatic terminal cancer should be treated with aggressive surgery that it is the morally right course or even that it is the best course.

It could well be that clinicians as a group have systematic evaluative biases that lead not only individual clinicians to favor such radical intervention, but also lead the group as a whole to have this distorted evaluation. Certain biases may have led them to enter the general field of medicine or their subspecialty of oncology in the first place. Those with abnormally high fear of cancer may have chosen oncology for their life's work.[10] Or systematic value orientations may be transmitted as part of the general socialization into the medical profession and its subspecialties. Clinicians are taught the particular Greek cultural worldview of the Hippocratic Oath as they learn their clinical roles. There is good reason to believe that clinicians developed the unique moral stance that supports benevolent lying to patients as part of their socialization into Hippocratic medicine.

The fact that there is a systematic evaluative consensus among a group of experts does not establish that that evaluation is correct. This is increasingly recognized in clinical medicine by, for example, the replacement of the professional standard with a reasonable (lay)person standard in the informed consent doctrine.[11] In court cases, such as the Quinlan case, we have seen that the professional consensus about preserving vegetative life was explicitly rejected in favor of a lay standard. For some reason, however, we have been slow to extend this conclusion to the public policy realm. Even when we have recognized the implication for policy questions, we have almost never considered the implications for the consensus of experts in developing a working presumption about what are believed to be scientific or medical facts.

CONSENSUS OF EXPERTS IN PUBLIC POLICY

The panels of experts assembled to deal with broad questions of public policy should raise the same problems as the use of groups of experts as clinical decision makers. At times the issues are addressed by relying on the distinction between facts and evaluations. The panels of experts proposed to function as "science courts," for example, are supposed to eschew all questions of value and address only matters of scientific fact.[12] Often overlooking the increasingly recognized difficulties of maintaining a rigid fact/value dichotomy, defenders of science courts in the 1970s insisted that the consensus of experts could at least be relied upon to provide the best possible statement of the scientific facts. Likewise, the *Participants' Guide to Consensus Development Conferences*, although apparently conceding that a pure fact/value separation is impossible, conceptualizes the task as essentially technical. It instructs, "The topic should be resolvable on technical grounds and the outcome should not depend mainly on the value judgments of panelists."[13]

In spite of this effort to create a role for expert consensus as a way of knowing factual matters, it is striking that many government panels of medical experts have been presented with lists of questions that naively mix clearly evaluative questions (such as whether the benefits of a technology exceed the risks and what the funding priorities ought to be) with matters that appear more like questions of scientific fact.

As we saw in the two previous chapters, the NIH consensus development panels have been notorious for their commingling of blatantly evaluative questions and those that appear more like matters of fact, about which scientifically trained experts in a particular field might be expected to possess expertise. Examples from the lists of charge questions given to the NIH panels include "What factors should be considered by the physician and patient in determining if and when ECT would be an appropriate treatment?"[14] and "Should an attempt be made to reduce the blood cholesterol levels of the general population?"[15] Clearly, deciding when ECT is appropriate involves judgments not only about the ethics of electroshock and compulsory treatment, but also comparisons about social priorities for funding. Deciding whether to launch an effort to lower blood cholesterol of the general population involves value judgments about the relative risks and benefits of blood cholesterol techniques (whether dietary changes are "worth it," for example) as well as decisions about funding priorities that, in principle, cannot be decided on the basis of the science alone. Another panel was asked, "What are the recommended forms of prophylaxis in [venous thrombosis and pulmonary embolism]?"[16] One cannot offer a recommendation on prophylaxis without incorporating judgments about the value of different interventions and their side effects, the use of resources for this purpose compared with other possible uses, and so forth.

Even more recent consensus conference reports contain blatant and controversial evaluative policy judgment. The statement on surgery for epilepsy, in response to the call for a value judgment about how outcome should be assessed, states that future studies ought to take into account "quality of life" as well as seizure control.[17] It explicitly makes the controversial, non-scientific judgment that effects on the well-being of the family and the society, as well of the patient, are legitimate criteria for evaluation of a surgical procedure.[18] In response to the call for a value judgment about how patients should be selected, the panel says we should limit surgery to cases in which medical and neurological treatments including antiepileptic drugs have had a reasonable trial.[19] Clearly, the choice between an attempt at surgery and antiepileptic drugs depends on some subtle, subjective judgments having to do with patient fear of surgery, repulsion with the chronic use of drugs, and so forth. There is good reason to suspect that surgeons and neurologists on the panel would each have systematic inclinations about such issues; however, it is the patient's inclination that is important, not the consensus of either the surgeons or the neurologists.

Deciding such policy questions requires knowledge not only of the science of the matter, but evaluative decisions about whether the risks and costs are worth it in comparison to other uses of resources, decisions about which experts in the circulatory system ought to have no special authority and about which they may, in fact, have special biases.

CONSENSUS OF EXPERTS TO ESTABLISH
SCIENTIFIC FACTS

No matter how controversial all that has been said thus far might sound to medical experts, public policy makers, and ordinary laypeople, I take it that it follows from some now rather standard applications of the insight that it is wrong to generalize expertise. One cannot presume that one is an expert in evaluating matters in an area simply because one is an expert in the science of the area. Moreover, to the extent that the experts in the area can be expected to hold values that vary systematically from the general public, we can expect that their clinical and policy recommendations will be systematically distorted in the direction of the special values.

All of this seems to follow from the classical affirmation of the fact/value dichotomy. That classical dichotomy has recently undergone reassessment, however. It is increasingly clear that the fact/value dichotomy cannot be maintained rigidly. As we have seen in the previous chapter, even the process of stating facts necessarily involves choices made on the basis of evaluation: selection of a conceptual scheme, the choice of which of an infinite set of possible observations are worth reporting, the selection of a level of statistical significance that will justify reaching a conclusion, and the selection of a set of statistical tests to be performed. Even if one acknowledges that there is an objective reality out there to be described, no finite human observer can give a value-free and concept-free account of that reality.

The point is not simply that real scientists are always fallible. The claim is more basic: Even if working as the ideal scientist, one must make evaluative and conceptual choices to present the facts in one's area of expertise.

The implications are radical. Rather sophisticated defenders of panels of experts have responded to the above "generalization of expertise" criticism by maintaining that panels of experts, such as those involved in the NIH consensus development panels, should rigorously limit their work to articulating the best possible estimates of the facts in the relevant area of expertise. They should not try to decide whether a radical mastectomy is better than a lumpectomy; they should limit their attention to reporting the survival rates from each procedure and other such apparently factual information, leaving to overt policy makers and patients the task of deciding what to do about the facts. They advocate what can be called the liberal solution to the question of the role of experts in the public policy process.

If, however, the critics of the fact/value dichotomy are correct, this liberal solution is doomed to fail; in theory it must fail. Conceptual and evaluative choices will necessarily shape how the facts are presented. To the extent that the groups of scientific experts have systematic value biases that shape their formulating and reporting of the facts, then even the consensus of the experts about the facts in a given area should be expected to be skewed. This is true even if they all practice their scientific craft perfectly and try as hard as possible to avoid bias or distortion.

A diagram may help clarify the picture. The top portion of figure 24.1 represents schematically the distribution of the views of recognized experts in a field about some important fact, such as the predicted five-year survival rate after a radical mastectomy. Notice that at the very beginning we will confront a controversy over who qualifies as an expert. Different medical subspecialists can be expected to have somewhat different views regarding any set of facts controversial enough to warrant assembling a panel of experts. Someone must decide who will represent the different subspecialties: medical oncologists, surgeons, epidemiologists, and so forth. This ignores the even larger controversies over others who claim expertise and who may have assessments of the facts that vary even more widely, say, practitioners

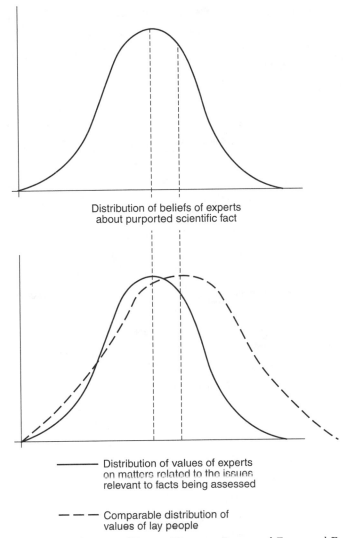

Distribution of beliefs of experts
about purported scientific fact

———— Distribution of values of experts
on matters related to the issues
relevant to facts being assessed

— — — Comparable distribution of
values of lay people

FIGURE 24.1 Distribution of Expert Views on Purported Facts, and Expert and Lay Views on Relevant Values.

of alternative healing methods such as Chinese medicine, holistic health, faith healing, and so forth.

It is not sufficient to solve the selection problem by choosing "one from each specialty." Do orthodox medicine and these alternative medicines each get one panel member? Surely not. Likewise, do oncologists, surgeons, and epidemiologists count as one group of experts (orthodox medicine) or do they count as three? Is there any reason to believe that they should be equally represented? Choosing who the panel members are will already partially predetermine the exact shape of the curve in figure 24.1.

Let us finesse that issue, however, and assume that we have a recognized group of experts on the survival rate following radical mastectomy and that their individual assessments produce the distribution curve at the top of the figure.

What policy makers want to know, of course, is which is the "real" survival rate. Finite scientists cannot answer that question. In the absence of an answer, there is a great temptation to take some average or consensus view of the experts as the best possible statement of the facts upon which policy judgments can be made. The thesis of this chapter is that there are solid theoretical reasons to hold that this average or consensus view of the experts is not the best estimate of the facts for making public policy.

We now know that among any group of experts, we can expect the conceptual and evaluative commitments of the individual members to vary somewhat. Moreover, the individual estimates of the scientific facts will vary with the evaluative and conceptual commitments.[20] In the example of radical mastectomy, we can expect evaluative variations that correlate with estimates of postmastectomy survival rates. Some will have a basic value orientation that is interventionist—for example, the surgeons who want to cut. Others will have atypical fear of cancer or unusual value commitments to the importance of maintaining the breast structure. All of these variations will create extremely complex value profiles among the experts. We can expect that different experts will report somewhat different estimates of survival rates and that these estimates will correlate with the value profiles of the individual scientists.

It is important to emphasize that this is not exclusively because scientists may be biased. In theory, even a perfect scientist would have to make evaluative and conceptual choices in defining the terms of the question being addressed, in choosing which data and which studies to emphasize, in selecting which data are important and which statistical tests are definitive. Even if these scientists on the panel of experts were entirely free of error, their estimates of the facts would correlate with their value profiles. In figure 24.1, their position on the top solid line curve (their beliefs about the facts) will correlate with their position on the bottom solid line curve (their values relevant to the facts being assessed).

Still, one might argue that the best estimate is the average or consensus estimate—that we should gravitate toward the center. There are serious theoretical problems with that position, however. First, social psychology tells us some intriguing things about consensus formation and group process.

In particular, the phenomenon known as *risky shift* takes place when groups are asked to make judgments. It has been shown that the consensus view of a group is not the same as the average of the preexisting views of the individuals who make up the group. Rather, there will be systematic and predictable shifts reflected in the consensus formation process.[21] Typically, the consensus of the group is more in favor of taking risks. If one could independently determine the view of each panel member and then take an average, the consensus of the group acting as a group would favor more risk taking than the average view of the individual members of the group.

More important, we can ask what the significance is of the known systematic differences between the general population's relevant values and the value profiles of the group of experts as a whole. Consider in figure 24.1 the dotted line curve, which represents a distribution of values of the general lay population to a policy such as endorsing or funding radical mastectomies. Presented schematically, we see in the diagram the representation that the value distribution of the general population is somewhat different from the group of experts. It has a different mean and a greater variance—both assumptions that are plausible and supported by empirical examples.

The critical question is, what facts would the general public choose as the basis for its public policy if, contrary to reality, it could be as educated as the experts about the relevant science? Possibly the process of becoming a expert in the relevant science would itself change the value profile in the direction of the values of the expert group, but I believe those making policy would reasonably want to know what estimate of the facts would be made by those holding the present values of the general public, but as knowledgeable as the experts about the scientific facts.

The answer can be read off the curves in figure 24.1. We can see that the consensus values of the general public (the mean or modal values in our diagram) are different from the consensus values of the experts. We can also determine what the estimate of the facts are of the expert who holds the values matching the consensus values of the general public. Once it is understood that the estimates of the facts by the experts should be expected to correlate with their value positions, it is hard to see why the public would want to use the set of consensus facts appropriate for those experts whose values they do not share. Laypeople should be more oriented to the estimate of the facts corresponding to the position on the curves of the experts who share the consensus values of the general public.

An example from outside of medicine may help clarify the point. Imagine a public trying to decide whether to build a nuclear power plant and realizing that it needed complex technical information about risks of an accident before making its final decision. Knowing that individual nuclear engineers might have idiosyncratic values that could influence projections of incidence rates, it might assemble a panel drawn from the most competent nuclear engineers available and take their consensus estimate of the risk of a particular defined event.

We can imagine, however, that at some earlier point there existed a pool of bright students deciding whether to enter the field of nuclear engineering. It seems reasonable that some would have values leading to low fears about nuclear energy whereas others would have values leading to high fears. It further seems reasonable that those with what could be called "antinuclear" values would choose other engineering specialties, leaving a pool of nuclear engineering experts whose values are systematically supportive of nuclear energy. The consensus values of actual nuclear engineers should be quite different from the consensus values of those who might have become nuclear engineers and chose to avoid the field. The consensus evaluations of the remaining experts ought to be atypical.

The same problem surely will occur when we rely on panels of medical experts to provide consensus estimates of the risks of a new medical technology. Imagine a public wanting to know, for example, what the risks were of gene therapy. They might assemble a panel of the world's leading experts in gene therapy technology and ask them to write a consensus report on the risks of producing genetic monstrosities, of releasing new genetic material into the species, of causing new diseases to be created, and so forth. A good panel would include some scientists who were unusually concerned about such risks and some scientists who minimized them. Knowing that individual scientists had idiosyncratic biases, we would create a panel covering a range of different perspectives. We would then be tempted to accept the average or consensus views about the risks as the best estimate—the estimate upon which we could base public policy.

That would be a mistake. Even bracketing the risky shift phenomenon, we should anticipate that some medical scientists would have self-selected themselves out of the pool of genetic scientists who were expert in gene therapy. They would choose to become urologists or experts in research on stomach ulcers. Some others might be so eager to engineer new human genetic forms that funders of research and those who hire medical professors would refuse to support them, forcing them out of the field. Those left to become experts in genetics would be a select group with unique values, probably more supportive of genetic engineering than the average member of the public. They would each have a unique genetic value profile. If their individual estimates of the likelihood of various catastrophic events occurring as a result of gene therapy are influenced by the value profiles and their value profiles are not the same as those of the typical member of the public, then the consensus estimate of the facts about various events occurring should be skewed.

Implications for the Use of Expert Consensus

If this is sound, the implications for the use of panels of experts in the public policy process are radical. Even for the task of providing unbiased estimates of facts upon which policy makers might later act, the answers given by panels of experts ought to reflect their consensus values and their consensus values ought to be different from those of the general public. Some strategies might be available for attempting to adjust for this seemingly necessary distortion.

MULTIPLE PANELS

One plausible strategy would be to arrange for multiple panels purposely structured based on the values of the experts constituting them. Presumably we would agree that competence should be a necessary condition for expertise (although there may be considerable dispute over what counts as competence). Among those considered competent, however, we might constitute a "liberal" and a "conservative" consensus panel, each kept blind to the deliberations of the other. The result would be two separate consensuses providing presumably differing estimates of the facts under question.

At least such a strategy should give some estimate of how sensitive the scientific judgments are to value considerations. If two panels deliberately constructed to represent conservative and liberal values reach essentially identical estimates of the facts, we can assume that they are dealing with a question relatively immune to the value distortions of concern. On the other hand, if they differ significantly, the policy maker at least knows the nature of the phenomenon being confronted.

SKEWED PANELS

Another strategy might be to stratify the sampling of experts so that it reflects the value distribution of the general public rather than the value distribution of the experts. As long as the panelists are selected from those recognized as experts and they undertake their task in the spirit of a scientific enterprise, the result should approach an estimate of the facts that would be made by the general public if only they had the scientific expertise of the panelists.

CORRECTING THE CONSENSUS

Still another possibility is letting the consensus panels work as they have in the past, generating consensuses about more factual questions, but recognizing that their report will predictably be distorted somewhat in the direction of the value consensus of the expert group and then making a political adjustment of the estimate of the facts to correct for this distortion. If a state legislature can establish that the public consensus values are more conservative about nuclear energy than the modal values of experts in nuclear engineering, it could self-consciously use a larger estimate of the risk than the consensus panel provides. It would not be irrational of unscientific to do so.

Political adjustments of the facts, however, must be seen as a dangerous enterprise. Surely, the policy makers would not want to overcompensate. They ought to want the most reliable estimate of the facts they can obtain. The point is that the most reliable estimate by those who are relatively antinuclear energy ought to be somewhat different from the most reliable estimate by those who are more in favor. There is absolutely no reason to assume that the average of the two biases is the most reliable set of facts upon which to base policy.

There may well be other strategies available for responding to this analysis of the use of consensus of expertise for establishing estimates of the facts. None of the strategies suggested is without its risks. The use of multiple panels is expensive and leaves open the theoretical question of how one ought to choose among conflicting estimates. The idea of skewing panel selection or purposely making a political adjustment of the facts seems heretical and poses dangers. Nevertheless, we must be aware that there are now good theoretical reasons why the consensus of experts about questions of purported fact as well as about evaluations ought to be seen as suspect. They will be suspect to the extent that the value distributions of the experts correlate with their estimates of the facts and differ systematically from those of the general population.

Epilogue

A Patient Manifesto

Patients of the world have too long suffered the plight of the passive. They have been told that "doctor knows best," and their job was to follow "doctor's orders." That may have made sense when people believed that deciding what was best was a matter of medical science, but it is foolishness that leads to oppression once we realize that it is impossible to know what is good for a patient without letting the patient make the value judgments.

Deciding what is best in literally every case requires a value judgment, and doctors can no longer be assumed to have any expertise in making those value judgments. Insofar as it is the patient's well-being that is at stake, the patient must be presumed to be the most likely to be the expert—the expert in deciding which among alternative expected outcomes is best for him or her. Patients need to know the current medical facts—facts about diagnosis, prognosis, and expected treatment outcomes. Physicians should continue to be presumed to be experts in this area (although even here physicians are often at the mercy of pharmaceutical company salespeople and biased presentation of data).

We must continue to expect the physician to provide us with the best possible diagnostic information, the most reasonable estimate of the expected outcome without treatment, and the plausible treatment options (including their likely effects). What physicians cannot do is tell their patients whether any particular outcome is good or bad. For one patient with a serious, perhaps fatal, illness, an aggressive, expensive treatment may offer real hope. The costs and the risks of sometimes terrible side effects may be worth it. But for another patient with the identical medical condition, the value judgments may be totally different. The risks may not be worth the candle.

Physicians have too long placed themselves in the position of priests with some sort of divine knowledge of what is good for patients. In fact, they have no basis for claiming such knowledge. They may even systematically make the wrong guesses about what is good for their patients.

The time has come to stop letting physicians impose their hunches about what is good for patients and start letting patients choose among the treatment options that are available. In a postmodern world of the new medicine:

1. The language of modern medicine is corrupting and must be abandoned.
    a. Doctors don't give orders. They provide their assessment of the medical facts and give evaluative advice if asked for it.
    b. Hospitals are not prisons. Patients are not discharged from them; they decide to leave, preferably upon the advice of various assistants acting as consultants. (Patients may be required to leave on the basis of institutional policy, but cannot be forced to stay and must not be required to "sign out against advice" if they decide to leave when the doctor's value judgment does not concur.)
    c. There is no such thing as a "medically indicated treatment." Medicines do not "indicate," and they can't be demonstrated to be good for someone except by means of a set of evaluative judgments that cannot be made adequately by physicians or by medical experts.
    d. No such thing as a "treatment of choice" exists except by the choice of the patient or the agent for the patient. The choice of a treatment by anyone else who does not have authority to make value judgments for the patient is a paternalistic imposition of someone else's values. Hence, no writer of a medical textbook and no panel of medical experts can determine that any particular treatment is the best. Treatments cannot legitimately be labeled as "treatments of choice."
    e. No treatment is ever "medically necessary." Any attempt to justify a treatment for insurance or legal purposes by claiming it is medically necessary is a confusion that merely hides the value judgments of the insurance company gatekeeper or the medical expert. No treatment is ever necessary (if one is willing to pay

the consequences of omitting it). No treatment is ever a luxury or unnecessary unless one has imposed a set of value judgments to reach this conclusion.

2. It is time to abandon informed consent. Consent was a welcome alternative to the more traditional unilateral imposition by a paternalistic physician onto a patient of his value judgments, but it is merely a halfway reform, a baby step toward the liberation of patients. Patients need choice, not consent to the physician's recommendations.

3. No longer can physicians justifiably prescribe medications for their patients. If they cannot know what is best, they cannot "prescribe" treatments. They should explain plausible options. They can educate patients about what the likely effects of the options are. They can even be called upon to certify that the patient understands adequately what the likely effects are. They cannot be gatekeepers who draw on their personal value judgments to decide which patients get access to chemicals and other treatments and which do not. If society needs to be protected, it is the values of the community through its representatives that must block public access to medications, not physicians whose values may match neither the patient's nor the public's. Patients should be given choices, not merely an opportunity to consent to the physician's options.

4. Patients can no longer be stigmatized by labels created by health professionals that classify them as acting immorally or irrationally if they make lifestyle choices that do not maximize their health. Longevity-maximizing lifestyles can be boring, painful, and irrational when they require sacrificing other nonmedical goods. Similarly, morbidity-minimizing lifestyles are not always the most reasonable in either the long or short run. It is not rational to maximize one's health when doing so comes at the expense of failing to maximize one's well-being. Thus, not all fat people are overweight. Not all skinny people are underweight. Physicians are not in a position to know whether people are at the weight that maximizes their well-being. They should not impose their private or biased health-maximizing value judgments on their patients. Many people are fat because they are rational.

5. Every person is entitled to a decent amount of health care funded through health insurance or government health services. Any single list of covered medical services will be a biased list conforming to the value judgments of those who make up the list, that is, the most powerful in the society. Those who are most marginal, those at the fringes, are likely to be in the least agreement with those value judgments

and are thus the victims of discrimination if they must have imposed upon them a single package of insured medical services. A decent amount of health care requires only that the cost of the insurance (adjusted for age) be the same for each person and that no one be excluded based on preexisting conditions that are beyond his or her control.

6. Hospice care is a right of every person at the end stage of life, but it is not medical care and should not be part of health insurance. It must be part of basic Social Security that is an entitlement of every member of the moral community. It should not be seen as merely medical, and its administration should not be dominated by health professionals.

7. People have a right not to have medical research conducted on them without their agreement or the agreement of their surrogate. They are entitled to high-quality medical science, including randomized clinical trials to determine the likely effects of various treatments, but no physician and no group of medical scientists can determine that the expected net benefits of two treatments are similar enough to justify randomizing patients in such trials. Only the willingness of the individual research subject to be randomized justifies such randomization. Potential subjects may have rational preferences for one treatment arm or the other, even if physicians or medical experts, based on their own values, are indifferent and thus in "equipoise." When they have a rational preference, subjects should have a right of access to the treatment of their preference provided access is not contrary to the public interest. Potential subjects may also be sufficiently indifferent to treatment alternatives that they agree to be randomly assigned one of them for the good of science even if physicians and medical experts have developed a preference for one of the treatments.

8. It is time to declare the end of the tyranny of the experts. Experts cannot determine that a treatment is either safe or effective without drawing on personally held values. Those values are likely to be biased and, in any case, not those that are shared by all patients. Judgments by the FDA, courts, medical review panels, insurance companies, and other gatekeepers based on the consensus of the experts reflect only the personal values of those experts, not a rational basis for limiting access to the ordinary patient.

9. Clinical practice guidelines, treatment protocols, and other bureaucratic mechanisms for telling physicians how to impose judgments on patients necessarily impose the value judgments of the writers on

patients and their physicians who endeavor to assist patients in making treatment choices. At best, they reflect how one should behave who holds the values of the writers. They do not necessarily reflect rational behavior for patients whose values are different.

10. Patients of the world, take responsibility for your own healing. You have nothing to lose but your passivity. Doctor no longer knows best.

NOTES

Notes to Introduction

1. In re Quinlan, 70 N.J. 10, 355 A. 2d 647 (1976), *cert. denied* sub nom., Garger v. New Jersey, 429 U.S. 922 (1976), overruled in part, In re Conroy, 98 NJ 321, 486 A.2d 1209 (1985).

2. I began seeing the moral offensiveness of the Hippocratic Oath in the early 1970s when I discovered that it failed to respect the rights of patients or of the surrounding society. See Robert M. Veatch, "Medical Ethics: Professional or Universal," *Harvard Theological Review* 65, no. 4 (October 1972):531–539; and later "The Hippocratic Ethic: Consequentialism, Individualism and Paternalism," in *No Rush to Judgment—Essays on Medical Ethics*, ed. David H. Smith and Linda M. Bernstein, 238–265 (Bloomington, IN: The Poynter Center, Indiana University, 1978); and "The Hippocratic Ethic Is Dead," *The New Physician* (September 1984):41–42, 48. These all represent essays in my evolution toward the discovery of the new medicine.

3. Ludwig Edelstein, "The Hippocratic Oath: Text, Translation and Interpretation," in *Ancient Medicine: Selected Papers of Ludwig Edelstein*, ed. Temkin, Owsei, and C. Lilian Temkin, 3–64 (Baltimore, MD: The Johns Hopkins Press, 1967).

4. Robert M. Veatch and Carol G. Mason, "Hippocratic vs. Judeo-Christian Medical Ethics: Principles in Conflict," *The Journal of Religious Ethics* 15 (Spring 1987): 86–105.

5. Paul Ramsey, *The Patient as Person* (New Haven, CT: Yale University Press, 1970).

Notes to Chapter 2

1. Robert M. Veatch, Amy Haddad, and Dan C. English, *Case Studies in Medical Ethics*, 2nd ed. (New York: Oxford, forthcoming).

2. The idea comes from Florence Rockwood Kluckhohn and Fred. L Strodtbeck, *Variations in Value Orientations* (Evanston, IL: Row, Peterson and Company, 1961).

3. A long time ago, I wrote a piece about this. Robert M. Veatch, "Doing What Comes Naturally," *Hastings Center Report* 1, no. 1 (September 1971):1–3.

Notes to Chapter 3

1. L. Edelstein, "The Hippocratic Oath: Text, Translation and Interpretation," *Ancient Medicine: Selected Papers of Ludwig Edelstein*, ed. O. Temkin and C. L. Temkin, 3–64 (Baltimore, MD: The Johns Hopkins Press, 1967), p. 6.
2. American Medical Association, Council on Ethical and Judicial Affairs, *Code of Medical Ethics: Current Opinions with Annotations, 1998–1999 Edition* (Chicago, IL: American Medical Association, 1998), p. 241.
3. H. Feifel et al., "Physicians Consider Death," in *Proceedings of the American Psychological Association* (1967), pp. 201–202.
4. A. R. Jonsen, "Do No Harm: Axiom of Medical Ethics," *Philosophical Medical Ethics: Its Nature and Significance*, ed. S. F. Spicker and H. T. Engelhardt, Jr., 27–41 (Boston, MA: D. Reidel, 1977); C. Sandulescu, "*Primum non nocere:* Philological Commentaries on a Medical Aphorism," *Acta Antiqua Hungarica* (1965) 13:359–368; R. M. Veatch, R. M., *A Theory of Medical Ethics* (New York: Basic Books, 1981), p. 161.
5. D. Parfit, "What Makes Someone's Life Go Best," *Reasons and Persons*, 493–503 (Oxford: Clarendon Press, 1984), pp. 493–494.
6. Ibid., p. 499.
7. R. M. Veatch, "Consensus of Expertise: The Role of Consensus of Experts in Formulating Public Policy and Estimating Facts," *The Journal of Medicine and Philosophy* 16 (1991):427–445.

Notes to Chapter 4

1. Fred Rosner and J. David Bleich, eds., *Jewish Bioethics* (New York: Sanhedrin Press, 1979).
2. B. M. Ashley and K. D. O'Rourke, *Healthcare Ethics: A Theological Analysis*, 3rd ed. (St. Louis, MO: The Catholic Health Association of the United States, 1989).
3. W. F. May, "Code, Covenant, Contract, or Philanthropy?" *Hastings Center Report* 5 (December 1975):29–38.
4. American Medical Association, 1975, "Principles of Medical Ethics of the American Medical Association [1903]," in T. Percival, *Percival's Medical Ethics, 1803*, reprint, ed. C. D. Leake, 240–257 (Baltimore, MD: Williams and Wilkins, 1975), p. 242.
5. Ibid., p. 243.
6. American Medical Association, Council on Ethical and Judicial Affairs, *Code of Medical Ethics: Current Opinions with Annotations, 1998–1999 Edition* (Chicago: American Medical Association, 1998), p. xiv.
7. Ibid, p. 135.
8. Immanuel Kant, "On the Supposed Right to Tell Lies from Benevolent Motives," *Critique of Practical Reason and Other Works on the Theory of Ethics*, trans. T. K. Abbott (London: Longmans, 1909 [1797]), 361–365.
9. W. D. Ross, *The Right and the Good* (Oxford: Oxford University Press, 1930).
10. "General Medical Council: Disciplinary Committee," *British Medical Journal Supplement* 3442 (March 20, 1971):79–80.
11. J. Kevorkian, *Prescription Medicide: The Goodness of Planned Death* (Buffalo, NY: Prometheus Books, 1991); T. Quill, *Death and Dignity: Making Choices and Taking Charge* (New York: Norton Press, 1993).

Notes to Chapter 5

1. D. H. Novack, B. J. Detering, R. Arnold, et al., "Physician's Attitudes toward Using Deception to Resolve Difficult Ethical Problems," *Journal of the American Medical Association*, 261, no. 20 (1989):2980–2985; also see E. H. Morreim, *Balancing Act: The New Medical Ethics of Medicine's New Economics* (Dordrecht, The Netherlands: Kluwer Academic Publishers, 1991).

2. Aristotle, *Nicomachean Ethics*, trans. M. Ostwald (Indianapolis, IN: Bobbs-Merrill, 1962), p. 119.

3. R. M. Veatch, "Justice and the Right to Health Care: An Egalitarian Account," in *Rights to Health Care*, ed. T. J. Bole III and W. B. Bondeson, 83–102 (Dordrecht, The Netherlands: Kluwer Academic Publishers, 1991).

4. E. L. Milford, L. Ratner, and E. Yunis, "Will Transplant Immunogenetics Lead to Better Graft Survival in Blacks?—Racial Variability in the Accuracy of Tissue Typing for Organ Donation: The Fourth American Workshop," *Transplantation Proceedings* 19 (Suppl. 2, April 1987):30–31.

5. W. D. Ross, *The Right and the Good* (Oxford: Oxford University Press, 1930).

6. Tom L. Beauchamp and James F. Childress, eds., *Principles of Biomedical Ethics*, 4th ed. (New York: Oxford University Press, 1994); Baruch Brody, *Life and Death Decision Making* (New York: Oxford University Press, 1988).

Notes to Chapter 7

1. Robert M. Veatch, *The Patient as Partner: A Theory of Human-Experimentation Ethics* (Bloomington, IN: Indiana University Press, 1987); Robert M. Veatch, *The Patient-Physician Relation: The Patient as Partner, Part 2* (Bloomington, IN: Indiana University Press, 1991).

2. Stuart J. Youngner, Wendy Lewandowski, Donna K. McClish, Barbara W. Juknialis, Claudia Coulton, and Edward T. Bartlett, "'Do Not Resuscitate' Orders," *Journal of the American Medical Association* 285 (1985):54–57; Susanna E. Bedell and Thomas L. Delbanco, "Choices about Cardiopulmonary Resuscitation in the Hospital: When Do Physicians Talk with Patients?" *The New England Journal of Medicine* 310, no. 17 (April 26, 1984):1089–1093.

3. Robert J. Levine, "Do Not Resuscitate Decisions and Their Implementation," *Dilemmas of Dying: Policies and Procedures for Decisions Not to Treat*, ed. Cynthia B. Wong and Judith P. Swazey, 23–41 (Boston: G. K. Hall Medical Publishers, 1981); Steven H. Miles, Ronald Cranford, and Alvin L. Schultz, "The Do-Not-Resuscitate Order in a Teaching Hospital," *Annals of Internal Medicine* 96 (May 1982):660–664.

4. President's Commission for the Study of Ethical Problems in Medicine and Biomedical and Behavioral Research, *Deciding to Forego Life-Sustaining Treatment: Ethical, Medical, and Legal Issues in Treatment Decisions* (Washington, DC: U.S. Government Printing Office, 1983).

Notes to Chapter 8

1. National Conference on Standards and Guidelines for Cardiopulmonary Resuscitation and Emerging Cardiac Care, "Standard and Guidelines for Cardiopulmo-

nary (CPR) and Emergency Cardiac Care (ECC)," *Journal of the American Medical Association* 255 (June 6, 1986):2980 [2905–2984] [italics added].

2. U.S. Department of Health and Human Services, "Child Abuse and Neglect Prevention and Treatment Program: Final Rule: 45 CFR 1340," *Federal Register: Rules and Regulations* 50, no. 72 (April 15, 1985):14878–14892 [p. 14887, italics added].

3. For more on the idea of a fact/value dichotomy, see W. Kohler, *The Place of Value in a World of Facts* (New York: Mentor Books, 1966); W. D. Hudson, *The Is/Ought Question* (London: MacMillan, 1969).

4. Edmund D. Pellegrino, "The Goals and Ends of Medicine: How Are They to Be Defined?" in *The Goals of Medicine: The Forgotten Issue in Health Care Reform*, ed. Mark J. Hanson and Daniel Callahan, 55–68 (Washington, DC: Georgetown University Press, 1999); Howard Brody and Franklin G. Miller, "The Internal Morality of Medicine; Explication and Application to Managed Care," *Journal of Medicine and Philosophy* 23 (1998):384–410; Edmund D. Pellegrino, "The Internal Morality of Clinical Medicine: A Paradigm for the Ethics of the Helping and Healing Professions," *Journal of Medicine and Philosophy* 26, no. 6 (2001):559–579.

5. Darrel W. Amundsen, "The Physician's Obligation to Prolong Life: A Medical Duty without Classical Roots," *Hastings Center Report* 8 (August 1978):23–30.

6. U.S. Department of Health and Human Services, "Child Abuse and Neglect Prevention and Treatment Program: Final Rule: 45 CFR 1340," *Federal Register: Rules and Regulations* 50, no. 72 (April 15, 1985):14888 [14878–14892].

Notes to Chapter 10

1. Another such transitional concept is the notion of *brain death*. In the 1970s it emerged as an alternative to more traditional heart-and-lung-oriented concepts of death, but even then scholars were beginning to doubt that the death of the entire brain—every last cell and function—had to be dead in order for a person to be dead. Now we speak of cerebral, cortical, neocortical, and "higher" brain death, as well as death based on whole brain criteria, leaving the term "brain death" almost meaningless.

2. Robert M. Veatch, "Three Theories of Informed Consent: Philosophical Foundations and Policy Implications," *The Belmont Report: Ethical Principles and Guidelines for the Protection of Human Subjects of Research* (Washington, DC: National Commission for the Protection of Human Subjects of Biomedical and Behavioral Research, DHEW Publication No. [05]78–0014), 26-1–26-66; President's Commission for the Study of Ethical Problems in Medicine and Biomedical and Behavioral Research, *Making Health Care Decisions: A Report on the Ethical and Legal Implications of Informed Consent in the Patient-Practitioner Relationship*, vol. 1 (Washington, DC: U.S. Government Printing Office, 1982); Ruth Faden and Tom L. Beauchamp in collaboration with Nancy N. P. King, *A History and Theory of Informed Consent* (New York: Oxford University Press, 1986); Jay Katz, *The Silent World of Doctor and Patient* (New York: The Free Press, 1984).

3. Ludwig Edelstein, "The Hippocratic Oath: Text, Translation and Interpretation," *Ancient Medicine: Selected Papers of Ludwig Edelstein*, ed. Owsei Temkin and C. Lilian Temkin, 3–64 (Baltimore, MD: The Johns Hopkins Press, 1967).

4. American Medical Association Council on Ethical and Judicial Affairs, *Code of Medical Ethics: Current Opinions with Annotations, 2006–2007* (Chicago, IL: AMA Press, 2006), p. 227.

5. Schloendorff v. New York Hospital (1914). In Jay Katz, *Experimentation with Human Beings: The Authority of the Investigator, Subject, Professions, and State in the Human Experimentation Process* (New York: Russell Sage Foundation, 1972), p. 526.

6. "Nuremberg Code, 1946," in *Encyclopedia of Bioethics*, vol. 4, ed. Warren T. Reich (New York: Free Press, 1978), pp. 1764–1765.

7. Based on Custody of a Minor Mass., 379 N.E. 2d 1053 (1978).

8. Robert M. Veatch, "Limits of Guardian Treatment Refusal: A Reasonableness Standard," *American Journal of Law and Medicine* 9, no. 4 (Winter 1984):427–468; Robert M. Veatch, *Death, Dying, and the Biological Revolution*, rev. ed. (New Haven, CT: Yale University Press, 1989).

9. Derek Parfit, "What Makes Someone's Life Go Best," *Reasons and Persons* (Oxford: Clarendon Press, 1984), pp. 493–503.

10. Ibid., p. 499; Bernard Gert, "Rationality, Human Nature, and Lists," *Ethics* 100 (1990):279–300.

11. Parfit, "What Makes Someone's Life Go Best," p. 499.

12. Gert, "Rationality, Human Nature, and Lists."

13. See David DeGrazia, "Value Theory and the Best Interests Standard," *Bioethics* 9 (1995):50–61.

Notes to Chapter 12

1. Because calling them "prescription drugs" begs the question of this chapter and calling them "ethical" is totally inappropriate, I will use the term "legend" drug to refer to these agents currently restricted to prescription access.

2. John Wesley, *Primitive Physick: or, An Easy and Natural Method of Curing Most Diseases*, 21st ed. (London: J Paramore, 1785), p. xi.

3. Jerry Menikoff, *Law and Bioethics: An Introduction* (Washington, DC: Georgetown University Press, 2001), pp. 356–357.

Notes to Chapter 13

1. Judith Areen, "The Legal Status of Consent Obtained from Families of Adult Patients to Withhold or Withdraw Treatment," *Journal of the American Medical Association* 258, no. 2 (July 10, 1987):229–235; Robert M. Veatch, "Limits of Guardian Treatment Refusal: A Reasonableness Standard," *American Journal of Law and Medicine* 9, no. 4 (Winter 1984):427–468.

2. Maureen L. Moore, "Their Life Is in the Blood: Jehovah's Witnesses, Blood Transfusions and the Courts," *Northern Kentucky Law Review* 10, no. 2 (1983):281–304; Yolanda V. Vorys, "The Outer Limits of Parental Autonomy: Withholding Medical Treatment from Children," *Ohio State Law Journal* 43, no. 3 (1981):813–829.

3. In the matter of Phillip Becker, 92 Cal. App. 3d 796, 156 Cal Rptr. 48 (1979), Cert. denied sub nom.; Bothman v. Warren B., 445 U.S. 949 (1980), p. 50.

4. H. Tristram Engelhardt, Stuart F. Spicker, and Bernard Towers, eds., *Clinical Judgment: A Critical Appraisal* (Dordrecht, Holland: D. Reidel, 1979).

Notes to Chapter 14

1. National Institutes of Health, National Heart, Lung, and Blood Institute, *Clinical Guidelines on the Identification, Evaluation, and Treatment of Overweight and Obesity in Adults—the Evidence Report* (Bethesda, MD: National Institutes of Health, 1998).
2. Ibid., p. 174.
3. Sirpa Sarlio-Lähteenkorva, Karri Silventoinen, and Eero Lahelma, "Relative Weight and Income at Different Levels of Socioeconomic Status," *American Journal of Public Health* 94, no. 3 (March 2004): 468–472.

Notes to Chapter 15

1. Jesper Lagergren, Reinhold Bergstrom, and Olf Nyren, "Association between Body Mass and Adenocarcinoma of the Esophagus and Gastric Cardia," *Annals of Internal Medicine* 130 (1999):883–890.
2. Dominique S. Michaud, Edward Giovannmucci, Walter C. Willett, Graham A. Colitz, Meir J. Stampfer, and Charles S. Fuchs, "Physical Activity, Obesity, Height, and the Risk of Pancreatic Cancer," *JAMA* 286 (2001):921–929.
3. Eugenia E. Calle, Carmen Rodriguez, Kimberly Walker-Thurmond, and Michael J. Thun, "Overweight, Obesity, and Mortality from Cancer in a Prospectively Studied Cohort of U.S. Adults," *New England Journal of Medicine* 348 (2003):1625–1638.
4. Tobias Kurth, Michael Gaziano, Klaus Berger, Carlos S. Kase, et al., "Body Mass Index and the Risk of Stroke in Men," *Archives of Internal Medicine* 162 (2002):2557–2561.
5. David B. Allison, Kevin R. Fontaine, JoAnn E. Manson, June Stevens, and Theodore B. VanItallie, "Annual Deaths Attributable to Obesity in the United States," *Journal of the American Medical Association* 282 (October 27, 1999):1530–1538. Although their title refers to "obesity," the authors base their calculations on those who are either overweight or obese (that is, those with a BMI of over 25 including those having a BMI under 30).
6. Katherine M. Flegal, Barry I. Graubard, David F. Williamson, and Mitchell H. Gail, "Excess Deaths Associated with Underweight, Overweight, and Obesity," *JAMA* 293 (2005):1861–1867.
7. Eugenia E. Calle, Michael J. Thun, Jennifer M. Petrelli, Carmen Rodriguez, and Clark W. Heath, "Body-Mass Index and Mortality in a Prospective Cohort of U.S. Adults," *New England Journal of Medicine* 341 (1999):1097–1105.
8. Kevin R. Fontaine, David T. Redden, Chenxi Wang, Andrew O. Westfall, and David B. Allison, "Years of Life Lost Due to Obesity," *JAMA* 289 (2003):187–193.
9. Flegal et al., "Excess Deaths Associated With Underweight, Overweight, and Obesity."
10. Timothy R. Wessel, Christopher B. Arant, Marian B. Olsen, B. Delia Johnson, et al., "Relationship of Physical Fitness vs Body Mass Index With Coronary Artery Disease and Cardiovascular Events in Women," *JAMA* 292 (2004): 1179–1187.
11. I. Sadaf Farooqi, Julia Keogh, Giles S. H. Yeo, Emma J. Lank, Tim Cheetham, and Stephen O'Rahilly, "Clinical Spectrum of Obesity and Mutations in the Melanocortin 4 Receptor Gene," *New England Journal of Medicine* 348 (2003):1085–1095.

12. For example, see "Gene Helps Trigger Obesity, Diabetes," *The Washington Post*, Nov. 14, 2000, p. A12.

13. 1. National Institutes of Health, National Heart, Lung, and Blood Institute, *Clinical Guidelines on the Identification, Evaluation, and Treatment of Overweight and Obesity in Adults—the Evidence Report* (Bethesda, MD: National Institutes of Health, 1998), p. 25.

14. As cited in ibid., p. 25.

15. As cited in ibid., p. 26.

16. As cited in ibid., p. 26.

17. Thorkild I., Sorensen, Rissanen, Aila, Korkeila Maarit, and Kaprio, Jaakko, "Intention to Lose Weight, Weight Changes, and 18-y Mortality in Overweight Individuals Without Co-morbidities," *PLoS Medicine* 2, no. 6 (June 2005):510–520, p. 510.

18. Ali H. Mokdad, Earl S. Ford, Barbara A. Bowman, William H. Dietz, Frank Vinicor, Virginia S. Bales, and James S. Marks, "Prevalence of Obesity, Diabetes, and Obesity-Related Health Risk Factors, 2001," *JAMA* 289 (2003):76–79.

19. Aviva Must, Jennifer Spadano, Eugenie H. Coakley, Alison E. Field, Graham Colditz, and William H. Dietz, "The Disease Burden Associated With Overweight and Obesity," *JAMA* 282 (October 27, 1999):1523–1530.

20. "Mortimer Adler Dies; Philosophy, Father of Great Books Program," *The Washington Post*, July 30, 2001, p. B7.

21. Linda Bacon, Judith S. Stern, Marta D. Van Loan, and Nancy L. Keim, "Size Acceptance and Intuitive Eating Improve Health for Obese, Female Chronic Dieters," *Journal of the American Dietetic Association* 105, no. 6 (June 2005):929–936.

22. Ibid., p. 936.

Notes to Chapter 16

1. Dan E. Beauchamp, "Universal Health Care, American Style: A Single Fund Approach to Health Care Reform," *Kennedy Institute of Ethics Journal* 2 (1992):125–135; Dan Beauchamp and Ronald L. Rouse, "Universal New York Health Care: A Single-Payer Strategy Linking Cost Control and Universal Access," *New England Journal of Medicine* 323 (1990):640–644.

2. Norman Daniels, *Just Health Care* (Cambridge, England: Cambridge University Press, 1985); President's Commission for the Study of Ethical Problems in Medicine and Biomedical and Behavioral Research, *Securing Access to Health Care*, vol. 1 (Washington, DC: U.S. Government Printing Office, 1983).

3. Paul Menzel, *Strong Medicine: The Ethical Rationing of Health Care* (New York: Oxford University Press, 1990).

4. Robert M. Veatch, "What Is a 'Just' Health Care Delivery?" in *Ethics and Health Policy*, ed. Robert M. Veatch and Roy Branson, 127–153 (Cambridge, MA: Ballinger, 1976).

Notes to Chapter 17

1. For a discussion of whether values are subjective or objective, see Derek Parfit, "What Makes Someone's Life Go Best," in *Reasons and Persons* (Oxford: Clarendon Press, 1984), pp. 493–503; Bernard Gert, "Rationality, Human Nature, and

Lists," *Ethics* 100 (1990):279–300; David DeGrazia, "Moving Forward in Bioethical Theory: Theories, Cases, and Specified Principlism," *Journal of Medicine and Philosophy* 17 (1992):511–539.

2. Ronald Dworkin, "What Is Equality? Part 2: Equality of Resources," *Philosophy and Public Affairs* 10 (1981):283–345; Robert M. Veatch, *The Foundations of Justice: Why the Retarded and the Rest of Us Have Claims to Equality* (New York: Oxford University Press, 1986).

3. Under a multiple-list plan (or a single list with optional supplemental insurance), a health-care provider would be under obligation only to deliver those services that are covered (perhaps supplemented by certain additional services that individuals are willing to self-fund). If providers are left with moral discomfort at treating two medically identical parties differently, they would be permitted to deliver additional services to those without coverage as acts of charity, but they should not confuse this situation with that arising when one patient has fair and adequate coverage and the other does not. With multiple lists, if a clinician were to fund a particular service by drawing on resources from the insurance plan of subscribers who have chosen not to fund that service, he or she should be seen as unfairly depriving others from their deserved resources.

4. Some who generally have been sympathetic to the multiple-list argument have claimed that those who manage or approve the lists should at least insist on excluding coverage for services that have not been proved effective. They want to exclude certain services on the basis of outcomes research, randomized clinical trials, and other research. For most lists that would probably also be the subscribers' desire, but such exclusions may create serious problems. Imagine, for example, a group of believers in laetrile, an extract of apricot pits that in the 1970s was believed by some to cure cancer. Some who believed in this alternative were willing to forgo orthodox chemotherapy, but insisted on including coverage for laetrile. Presumably these are people who remained unpersuaded by the available evidence that orthodox chemotherapy may work and that laetrile will not. These are people who would decline chemotherapy, seeing it as worthless given their values and beliefs, but were terribly distraught if they could not gain access to the laetrile. Is there any moral reason why, if properly informed, they should not be permitted to spend their pooled insurance entitlement on something that they believe will increase their well-being more than alternative uses of their entitlement? As long as they can fund the desired, unproven remedy and it does not harm third parties, real defenders of the multiple-list idea would permit a group of laetrile believers to form and, provided there is a large enough group to make the group workable, let them forgo orthodox therapy in favor of spending their resources on something that they believe will buy them more quality-adjusted life years.

5. Robert M. Veatch, "The Ethics of Promoting Herd Immunity," *Family and Community Health* 10, no. 1 (1987):44–52.

6. Norman Daniels, *Am I My Parents' Keeper?: An Essay on Justice Between the Young and the Old* (New York: Oxford University Press, 1988).

7. It should be clear that the arguments put forward here for a multiple-list approach would also apply to other health-care systems that are not based on single payers or even on universal coverage. I take it to be uncontroversial that if a society

adopts a multiple-payer, free-market system of health insurance, multiple lists of services will be an inherent part of the system. The purpose of this chapter has been to show that the multiple-list approach is defensible, indeed necessary, for a fair and efficient single-payer system.

Notes to Chapter 18

1. Darrel W. Amundsen, "The Physician's Obligation to Prolong Life: A Medical Duty without Classical Roots," *Hastings Center Report* 8 (August 1978):23–30.
2. In the Matter of Baby K, 1993 WL 343557 (E.D. Va.); In re Jane Doe, a minor, civil Action File No. D-93064, Superior Court of Fulton County, State of Georgia, October 1991; In Re The Conservatorship of Helga Wanglie, State of Minnesota, District Court, Probate Court Division, County of Hennepin, Fourth Judicial District, June 28, 1991; Rideout, Administrator of Estate of Rideout, et al. v. Hershey Medical Center, Dauphin County Report, 1995, pp. 472–498; Velez v. Bethune et al. 466 S.E. 2d 627 (Ga. App. 1995); Gina Kolata, "Withholding Care from Patients: Boston Case Asks Who Decides," *New York Times* April 3, 1995, pp. A1, B8.
3. Sandol Stoddard, *The Hospice Movement: A Better Way of Caring for the Dying*, rev. ed. (New York: Vintage Books, 1992), p. 10.
4. Ibid., p. 11.
5. Shirley Du Boulay, *Cicely Saunders Founder of the Modern Hospice Movement* (New York: Amaryllis Press, 1984).
6. Ibid., pp. 156–157.
7. Cicely Saunders, "A Personal Therapeutic Journey," *British Medical Journal* 313 (1996):1599–1601.
8. Ibid.
9. Ibid.
10. Ibid., p. 1600.
11. M. J. Friedrich, "Hospice Care in the United States: A Conversation with Florence S. Wald," *Journal of the American Medical Association* 281 (1999):1683–1685, p. 1684.

Notes to Chapter 19

1. Reportedly, many other musicians famous in the field of bluegrass eventually would stop by, sometimes playing for the master. The visitors included Marty Stuart, Johnny Cash, Del McCoury, Kathy Chiavola, Ricky Skaggs, and former Blue Grass Boys Butch Robbins, Roland White, Mac Wiseman, and Tater Tate. See Richard D. Smith, *Can't You Hear Me Callin': The Life of Bill Monroe, Father of Bluegrass* (Boston: Little, Brown and Company, 2000), pp. 284–285.
2. Nicky James and David Field, "The Routinization of Hospice: Charisma and Bureaucratization," *Social Science and Medicine* 34 (1992):1363–1375.

Notes to Chapter 20

1. Murray W. Enkin, "Clinical Equipoise and Not the Uncertainty Principle Is the Moral Underpinning of the Randomised Controlled Trial," *BMJ* 321 (September

23, 2000):757–758; R. Peto and C. Baigent, "Trials: The Next 50 Years," *BMJ* 317 (1998):1170–1171; R. Peto, M. C. Pike, P. Armitage, N. E. Breslow, D. R. Cox, S. V. Howard, et al., "Design and Analysis of Randomized Clinical Trials Requiring Prolonged Observation of Each Patient. I. Introduction and Design," *British Journal of Cancer* 34 (1976):585–612.

2. Robert M. Veatch, *The Patient as Partner—A Theory of Human-Experimentation Ethics* (Bloomington, IN: Indiana University Press, 1987), pp. 210–211.

3. Charles Fried, *Medical Experimentation: Personal Integrity and Social Policy* (New York: American Elsevier, 1974), pp. 51–52; Benjamin Freedman, "Equipoise and the Ethics of Clinical Research," *New England Journal of Medicine* 317, no. 3 (1987):141–145; Charles Weijer, "Clinical Equipoise and Not the Uncertainty Principle Is the Moral Underpinning of the Randomised Controlled Trial," *BMJ* 321 (September 23, 2000):756–757.

4. In fact, it is increasingly clear that there are many reasons why the old Hippocratic ethic must be abandoned. It conflicts in many important ways with both religious and secular ethics that are plausible. Doing what the physician believes will benefit the patient requires ignoring all interests of all other parties; it requires ignoring any autonomous choices that patients make; it requires ignoring any rights-claims of patients or any deontological duties that physicians might have; and it requires paternalistically ignoring the patient's interpretation of what is in the patient's interest. No rational person, physician or layperson, would today follow the Hippocratic principle. For further explication of the problems with Hippocratic ethics see my articles "The Hippocratic Ethic: Consequentialism, Individualism and Paternalism," in *No Rush to Judgment—Essays on Medical Ethics*, ed. David H. Smith and Linda M. Bernstein, 238–265 (Bloomington, IN: The Poynter Center, Indiana University, 1978); [with Carol G. Mason] "Hippocratic Vs. Judeo-Christian Medical Ethics: Principles in Conflict," *The Journal of Religious Ethics* 15 (Spring 1987):86–105; and "Doctor Does Not Know Best: Why in the New Century Physicians Must Stop Trying to Benefit Patients," *Journal of Medicine and Philosophy*, forthcoming; as well as *A Theory of Medical Ethics* (New York: Basic Books, 1981).

5. A major dispute is currently raging about the moral acceptability of using placebos in cases in which an experimental treatment is to be tested and a standard therapy exists. See Richard Woodman, "Storm Rages Over Revisions to Helsinki Declaration," *BMJ* 319 (Sept. 11, 1999):660; Brian Vastag, "Helsinki Discord? A Controversial Declaration," *JAMA* 284 (Dec. 20, 2000):2983–2985. The World Medical Association's Declaration of Helsinki (World Medical Association, "Declaration of Helsinki—1964, revised 1975, 1983, and 1989," in *Encyclopedia of Bioethics*, rev. ed., vol. 5., ed. Warren T. Reich [New York: Simon & Schuster Macmillan, 1995], pp. 2765–2767; World Medical Association, "Declaration of Helsinki: Ethical Principles for Medical Research Involving Human Subjects," *JAMA* 284 [Dec. 20, 2000]:3043–3045) insists that the best available therapy must be made available, which seems to imply that in such cases, a placebo is unethical (Kenneth J. Rothman, Karin B. Michels, and Michael Baum, "For and Against: Declaration of Helsinki Should Be Strengthened," *British Medical Journal* 321 [August 12, 2000]:442–445). Part of the controversy has to do with

whether there is a known effective therapy "available" if it is on the market and used in the developed world but unavailable for economic reasons in the developing world. See Peter A. Clark, "The Ethics of Placebo-Controlled Trials for Perinatal Transmission of HIV in Developing Countries," *Journal of Clinical Ethics* 9, no. 2 (1998):156–166; Robert J. Levine, "The 'Best Proven Therapeutic Method' Standard in Clinical Trials in Technologically Developing Countries," *Journal of Clinical Ethics* 9, no. 2 (1998):167–172. Independent of that controversy is a line of argument that purports to defend the use of a placebo control in certain cases even if a known available therapy is available. Robert Temple and Susan S. Ellenberg ("Placebo-Controlled Trials and Active-Control Trials in the Evaluation of New Treatments: Part 1: Ethical and Scientific Issues," *Annals of Internal Medicine* 133, no. 6 [2000]:455–463; "Placebo-Controlled Trials and Active-Control Trials in the Evaluation of New Treatments: Part 2: Practical Issues and Specific Cases," *Annals of Internal Medicine* 133, no. 6 [2000]:464–470) have claimed that there are important scientific reasons in some cases to use a placebo control. They acknowledge that it would be unethical to randomize an experimental agent against a placebo if serious, long-term harm could be done by forgoing a standard therapy known to be effective, but defend the moral legitimacy of using a placebo when necessary if omitting the standard treatment will not cause permanent harm and the subject gives adequate consent. They cite situations in which a patient might temporarily forgo an analgesic for a headache as an example.

Temple and Ellenberg seem to be right at least in theory. Asking a subject to make a small, temporary sacrifice for the good of science is not immoral. It is conceptually similar to asking a normal healthy subject to take a small risk for the good of science (submitting to a draw of a small amount of blood, for example). In fact, although Temple and Ellenberg seem to categorically exclude cases in which the subject would be at risk of permanent harm by submitting to a placebo, it seems that not even all of these cases should be excluded. For example, a patient who, after considering a standard chemotherapy protocol, finds that the projected benefits outweigh the risks only ever so slightly, might legitimately be asked to forgo that expected benefit and agree to be randomized in a manner in which he risks getting a placebo. If the net benefit was seen by the patient as having a small enough advantage over the placebo (so small that the patient would have to struggle in doing the balancing to determine that the net expected result was a plus), it is hard to see how this case differs from the aspirin versus placebo example. What is critical is that the subject is not being asked to give up very much, not that the failure to receive the standard treatment involved a risk of permanent harm.

The only problem raised by the view of Temple and Ellenberg is that this rationale for the inclusion of placebos may prove so tempting to investigators that it could be abused. Because it may be cheaper and easier to show a difference between a new drug and a placebo, investigators and their funding agents may be tempted to argue for the placebo-controlled trial. The other reason that Temple and Ellenberg's position has been seen as controversial is that some of their critics have failed to perceive that they are excluding cases in which there are serious risks of harm if a placebo group is included. They sometimes sound as if they are insisting on randomization against placebo(s) in all cases. This is clearly a misreading of their position (even if they occasionally invite the criticism).

6. I will not pursue here the controversial question of whether a request to a competent patient to take a large risk for the good of science would be morally justified if the patient were adequately informed and freely consented to that large risk.

7. This distinction between absolute and approximate indifference is similar to Benjamin Freedman's distinction between *theoretical* and *clinical* equipoise. I think my terms are clearer. See Benjamin Freedman, "Equipoise and the Ethics of Clinical Research."

8. There may, of course, be other moral conditions imposed on research beyond approximate indifference and consent. For example, there needs to be equity in subject selection. There also needs to be adequate protection of privacy, and so forth. The point here is that approximate indifference along with adequate consent seems to be a necessary condition for justified research.

9. For purposes of this chapter I will not distinguish between the clinicians and the medical scientists. It is, of course, possible—I would suggest, probable—that those who primarily care for patients will have different evaluations of the costs and benefits of the therapies under consideration. If something important were eventually to determine whether it was the equipoise or indifference of the clinicians or the scientists that counted, this matter would have to be pursued. I shall suggest later in this chapter, however, that neither of them is definitive, so I will not agonize over the difference between the two.

10. Freedman, "Equipoise and the Ethics of Clinical Research." For a more recent defense of this view, see Charles Weijer, "Clinical Equipoise and Not the Uncertainty Principle Is the Moral Underpinning of the Randomized Controlled Trial," *BMJ* 321 (September 23, 2000):756–757.

11. Freedman, "Equipoise and the Ethics of Clinical Research," p. 141.

12. Ibid. Freedman gives an example of doubt within a scientific community over which of two treatments produces a greater survival rate. If there is equivalent evidence for alternative hypotheses, then we might say that the question is in doubt scientifically.

13. Ibid.

14. Benjamin Freedman, "Placebo-Controlled Trials and the Logic of Clinical Purpose," *IRB: A Review of Human Subjects Research* 40, no. 6 (1990):1–6.

15. To make matters more complex, Gifford uses the theoretical/clinical language not exactly in the same way that Freedman does. Gifford sometimes uses this language to refer to the difference between equipoise regarding the scientific question and equipoise regarding the clinical question. He, however, also uses it to refer to whether the standard is "fastidious" (more or less what Freedman has in mind when he speaks about the community being "exactly balanced") or is "pragmatic" (more or less what Freedman means when he speaks of a "lack of consensus in the clinical community" even though that community may not be exactly balanced). See Fred Gifford, "Freedman's 'Clinical Equipoise' and 'Sliding Scale All-Dimensions-Considered Equipoise,'" *Journal of Medicine and Philosophy* 25 (2000):400. Rather than the two distinctions outlined by Gifford, the situation is

even more complex. There are, in fact, at least three different distinctions: between individual and community equipoise, between equipoise on a scientific question and equipoise (indifference) on the question of the value of treatment options, and between the community being exactly balanced and it lacking a consensus even though it may not be exactly balanced. Gifford himself later notes these complexities (p. 408). I shall argue that, in the end, none of the subtle distinctions made by Freedman and Gifford make any difference in the justification of randomization.

16. I have spent a career arguing that even the factual determinations of science inevitably incorporate judgments about concepts and values. It is not that the scientist will inevitably be biased, but that even the ideal scientists cannot be value free. Nevertheless, we can ignore this problem for most of what is said about the more obvious evaluative judgments necessary to determine that two expected treatment outcomes are of approximately equal value. See Robert M. Veatch, *Value-Freedom in Science and Technology* (Missoula, MT: Scholars Press, 1976); and Robert M. Veatch and William E. Stempsey, "Incommensurability: Its Implications for the Patient/Physician Relation," *Journal of Medicine and Philosophy* 20, no. 3 (June 1995):253–269.

17. Several contributors to the debate have all helped sort out these problems. See Fred Gifford, "Community-Equipoise and the Ethics of Randomized Clinical Trials," *Bioethics* 9, no. 2 (1995):127–148; Fred Gifford, "Freedman's 'Clinical Equipoise'"; Jason H. T. Karlawish and John Lantos, "Community Equipoise and the Architecture of Clinical Research," *Cambridge Quarterly of Healthcare Ethics* 6, no. 4 (1997):385–396; and Richard Ashcroft, "Equipoise, Knowledge and Ethics in Clinical Research and Practice," *Bioethics* 13, no. 3–4 (1999):314–326; Richard Ashcroft, "Giving Medicine a Fair Trial," *BMJ* 320 (June 24, 2000):1686.

18. Robert M. Veatch, "Longitudinal Studies, Sequential Design, and Grant Renewals: What to Do with Preliminary Data," *IRB* (June/July 1979):1–3. See also Robert M. Veatch, *The Patient as Partner*.

Notes to Chapter 21

1. There are interesting special cases in which the scientific or clinical community believes a scientific question is settled, yet the lay community remains in doubt. The clinical effectiveness of laetrile (an extract of apricot pits) in curing cancer is an example. The clinical community was overwhelmingly convinced this extract was useless in curing cancer, yet there was widespread public belief it might be effective. Undertaking a carefully controlled clinical trial among willing, informed volunteers might be justified to resolve the matter in the minds of the lay population, even though the scientific community had no doubt about the outcome.

2. Of course, a wise lay population will factor in the eventual value of more theoretical knowledge. Even then, however, it is not "knowledge for the sake of knowledge." Rather, it is "knowledge for the sake of its unknown, but hoped for, uses."

3. The term "more or less" is taken here to cover the possibility, discussed earlier in this analysis, that even though the subject has a preference for one of the treatment arms and thus deviates from his or her personal indifference point, that subject is willing to forgo any perceived advantage for the good of science.

4. Robert M. Veatch, "Justice and Research Design: The Case for a Semi-Randomized Clinical Trial," *Clinical Research* 31 (February 1983):12–22. There are exceptions to my general conclusion that because permitting nonrandomized access is better science, persons preferring the experimental treatment should have access to it within the protocol. If a treatment is inherently scarce or granting access jeopardizes access to randomized patients, then access could be limited. Also, clinicians and manufacturers should have a limited right of conscience to refuse to provide treatments to patients. Also, even if the patient rationally prefers a treatment, the clinician who finds it offensive has some right not to provide it, at least if he can refer the patient to another provider. My conclusion for purposes of this article is merely that because she is not indifferent between the two treatments, one cannot rely on arguments from indifference or equipoise to justify randomizing her. If the treatment she prefers is available outside the protocol or if it can be provided in the protocol without jeopardizing the research, then it should be made available. The investigators cannot claim that granting her access is contrary to her interests because they themselves have accepted the null hypothesis as the moral foundation for the randomization.

5. I have elsewhere called this the "preliminary data problem." See Robert M. Veatch, "Longitudinal Studies, Sequential Design, and Grant Renewals: What to Do with Preliminary Data," *IRB* (June/July 1979):1–3.

6. Julia A. Pedroni, *Moral Problems in the Monitoring of Clinical Trial Data and Access to Interim Results* (doctoral dissertation, Georgetown University, Washington, DC), 1998.

7. Ruth Faden and Tom L. Beauchamp in collaboration with Nancy N. P. King, *A History and Theory of Informed Consent* (New York: Oxford University Press, 1986), pp. 256–262.

Notes to Chapter 22

1. The very term *manage* is controversial. It is used repeatedly in the technology assessment literature, particularly by the Agency for Health Care Policy and Research (AHCPR) *Clinical Practice Guidelines*, which uses the term in many of its titles. See such titles as *Management of Contract in Adults* and *Diagnosing and Managing Unstable Angina*. The imagery of managing a human being is considered offensive by some critics of contemporary health care who believe it implies a paternalism, a lack of respect for patient autonomy, yet the writers of these guidelines appear not to grasp this controversy. It is pejorative in the same way that *girl* is when used to refer to adult females or *boy* to refer to African-African American adult males. To these critics, management is something one does to a commodities portfolio or a group of subordinate employees.

2. Robert M. Veatch, "Values in Routine Medical Decisions" and "The Concept of 'Medical Indications,'" in *The Patient-Physician Relation: The Patient as Partner, Part 2* (Bloomington, IN: Indiana University Press, 1991), pp. 47–62.

3. P. C. Albertsen, J. H. Wasson, and M. J. Barry, "Observation as a Treatment Option among Men with Clinically Localized Prostate Cancer," in *Prostate Cancer* (New York: Wiley-Liss), pp. 185–196, cited in "PORT Researchers Discuss

Treatment Options and Use of Serum PSA Screening to Detect Prostate Cancer," *Research Activities* 181 (January 1995):5.

4. Office for Medical Applications of Research, *Participants' Guide to Consensus Development Conferences* (Bethesda, MD: U.S. Department of Health, Education, and Welfare, n.d.), p. 1.

5. NIH Consensus Development Panel on Gallstones and Laparoscopic Cholecystectomy, "Gallstones and Laparoscopic Cholecystectomy," *JAMA* 269, no. 8 (1993): 1018–1024, p. 1021.

6. Ibid., p. 1019.

7. National Institutes of Health, "Consensus Development Conference Statement: Dental Sealants in the Prevention of Tooth Decay," *Journal of Dental Education* 48, Supplement, (February 1984):126–131.

8. Robert F. Nease et al., "Variation in Patient Utilities for Outcomes of the Management of Chronic Stable Angina: Implications for Clinical Practice Guidelines," *JAMA* 273, no. 15 (1995):1185–1190.

9. Agency for Health Care Policy and Research, Public Health Service, U.S. Department of Health and Human Services, *Management of Cataract in Adults,* no. 4 (Washington, DC: U.S. Government Printing Office, 1994).

10. Agency for Health Care Policy and Research, Public Health Service, U.S. Department of Health and Human Services, *Management of Cancer Pain: Adults*, no. 9 (Washington, DC: U.S. Government Printing Office, 1994), pp. 8–9.

11. Agency for Health Care Policy and Research, Public Health Service, U.S. Department of Health and Human Services, *Depression in Primary Care: Detection, Diagnosis, and Treatment*, Quick Reference Guide for Clinicians, no. 5 (Washington, DC: U.S. Government Printing Office, 1993), p. 6.

12. Agency for Health Care Policy and Research, Public Health Service, U.S. Department of Health and Human Services, *Managing Otitis Media with Effusion in Young Children*, no. 12 (Washington, DC: U.S. Government Printing Office, 1994), p. 6.

13. Ibid., p. 5.

14. Robert M. Veatch, "Abandoning Informed Consent," *Hastings Center Report* 25, no. 2 (1995):5–12.

15. Judith Areen, "The Legal Status of Consent Obtained from Families of Adult Patients to Withhold or Withdraw Treatment," *Journal of the American Medical Association* 258, no. 2, (1987):229–235; Robert M. Veatch, "Limits of Guardian Treatment Refusal: A Reasonableness Standard," *American Journal of Law and Medicine* 9, no. 4 (1984):427–468.

16. For some public policy purposes, the proper values may not be those of the individual patient; they may be those of the society, but the values of the clinician still cannot legitimately come into play.

Notes to Chapter 23

1. "AHCPR Invites Proposals for PORT-II Projects," *Research Activities* 167 (August 1993):15.

2. "Ischemic Heart Disease PORT Publishes Latest Findings," *Research Activities* 176 (July 1994):6–7.

3. Ibid., p. 6.

4. C. Fleming et al., "A Decision Analysis of Alternative Treatment Strategies for Clinically Localized Prostate Cancer," *JAMA* 269, no. 20 (1993):2650–2658.

5. See National Institutes of Health, Office for Medical Applications of Research. *Participants' Guide to Consensus Development Conferences* (Bethesda, MD: U.S. Department of Health, Education, and Welfare, n.d.), in which one of the stated criteria for the conferences is "The topic should be resolvable on technical grounds and the outcome should not depend manly on value judgments of panelists."

6. National Institutes of Health Consensus Development Panel, "Critical Care Medicine," *JAMA* 250, no. 6 (1983):798–804.

7. Office for Medical Applications of Research, "Electroconvulsive Therapy," *JAMA* 254, no. 15 (1985):2103–2108.

8. Office for Medical Applications of Research, "Lowering Blood Cholesterol to Prevent Heart Disease," *JAMA* 253, no. 14 (1985):2080–2086.

9. Ludwig Fleck, *Genesis and Development of a Scientific Fact*, ed. Thaddeus J. Trenn and Robert K. Merton, trans. Fred Bradley and Thaddeus J. Trenn (Chicago: University of Chicago Press, 1979).

10. Thomas S. Kuhn, *The Structure of Scientific Revolutions* (Chicago: University of Chicago Press, 1962).

11. P. K. Feyerabend, *Realism, Rationalism & Scientific Method: Philosophical Papers, Volume* 1 (Cambridge: Cambridge University Press, 1981).

12. Peter L. Berger and Thomas Luckmann, *The Social Construction of Reality* (New York: Doubleday, 1967).

13. Robert M. Veatch, *Value-Freedom in Science and Technology* (Missoula, MT: Scholars Press, 1976). For some public policy purposes, the proper values may not be those of the individual patient; they may be those of the society.

14. Kuhn, 1962.

15. Veatch, *Value-Freedom in Science and Technology*.

Notes to Chapter 24

1. President's Commission for the Study of Ethical Problems in Medicine and Biomedical and Behavioral Research, *Making Health Care Decisions: A Report on the Ethical and Legal Implications of Informed Consent in the Patient-Practitioner Relationship*, vol. 1 (Washington, DC: U.S. Government Printing Office, 1982).

2. National Institutes of Health Consensus Development Panel, "Critical Care Medicine," Journal of the American Medical Association 250 (1983):798–804.

3. OMAR (Office of Medical Applications of Research), "Defined Diets and Childhood Hyperactivity," *Journal of the American Medical Association* 248 (1982): 290–292.

4. OMAR, "Consensus Statement on Mood Disorders: Pharmacologic Prevention of Recurrences," *Journal of the American Medical Association* 252 (1984):1264.

5. National Institutes of Health, "Consensus Development Conference Statement: Dental Sealants in the Prevention of Tooth Decay," *Journal of Dental Education* 48 (Supplement) (1984):126–131.

6. OMAR, *Coronary Artery Bypass Surgery*, NIH Consensus Development Conference Summary, vol. 3, no. 8 (Bethesda, MD: U.S. Department of Health and Human Services, n.d.).

7. OMAR, *NIH Consensus Development Conferences 1977–1978* (Bethesda, MD: U.S. Department of Health, Education, and Welfare, 1979); OMAR, *Consensus Development Conference Summaries, Volume 2, 1979* (Bethesda, MD: U.S. Department of Health, Education, and Welfare, 1980); OMAR, *Consensus Development Conference Summaries, Volume 3, 1980* (Bethesda, MD: U.S. Department of Health, Education, and Welfare, 1981); OMAR, *NIH Consensus Development* (Bethesda, MD: U.S. Department of Health and Human Services, n.d.); OMAR, *Participants' Guide to Consensus Development Conferences* (Bethesda, MD: U.S. Department of Health, Education, and Welfare, n.d.).

8. In re Quinlan, 70 N.J. 10, 355 A. 2d 647 (1976), *cert. denied* sub nom., Garger v. New Jersey, 429 U.S. 922 (1976), overruled in part, In re Conroy, 98 NJ 321, 486 A.2d 1209 (1985).

9. R. M. Veatch, "Generalization of Expertise: Scientific Expertise and Value Judgments," *Hastings Center Studies* 1, no. 2 (1973):29–40.

10. H. Feifel et al., "Physicians Consider Death," *Proceedings of the American Psychological Association* (1967):201–202.

11. Ruth Faden and T. L. Beauchamp in collaboration with N. P. King, *A History and Theory of Informed Consent* (New York: Oxford University Press, 1986); P. S. Appelbaum, C. W. Lidz, and A. Meisel, *Informed Consent: Legal Theory and Clinical Practice* (New York: Oxford University Press, 1987); Cobbs v. Grant, 1972, 502 P.2d 1 (Cal.); Canterbury v. Spence, 1972, 464 F. 2d 772 (D.C. Cir.).

12. R. E. Talbott, "'Science Court': A Possible Way to Obtain Scientific Certainty for Decisions Based on Scientific 'Fact'?" *Environmental Law* 8 (1978):827–850; J. A. Martin, "The Proposed Science Court," *Michigan Law Review* 75 (1977):1058–1091; B. M. Casper, "Technology, Policy and Democracy: Is the Proposed Science Court What We Need?" *Science* 194 (1976):29–35.

13. OMAR, *Participants' Guide to Consensus Development Conferences* (Bethesda, MD: U.S. Department of Health, Education, and Welfare, n.d.).

14. OMAR, "Electroconvulsive Therapy," *Journal of the American Medical Association* 254 (1985a):2103–2108.

15. OMAR, "Lowering Blood Cholesterol to Prevent Heart Disease," *Journal of the American Medical Association* 253 (1985b):2080–2086.

16. OMAR, "Prevention of Venous Thrombosis and Pulmonary Embolism," *Journal of the American Medical Association* 256 (1986a):744–749.

17. OMAR, "Surgery for Epilepsy," *Journal of the American Medical Association* 264 (1990):731.

18. Ibid., p. 732.

19. Ibid., p. 730.

20. R. M. Veatch, *Value-Freedom in Science and Technology* (Missoula, MT: Scholars Press, 1976).

21. C. Fraser et al., "Risky Shifts, Cautious Shifts and Group Polarization," *European Journal of Social Psychology* 1 (1971):7–30.